CONFERENCE PROCEEDINGS OF NATIONAL CONFERENCE ON COMPUTATIONAL ADVANCEMENTS IN RESEARCH AND EDUCATION FOR PHARMACEUTICAL EXCELLENCE (CARE 2024)

Organized by

Aditya Group of Pharmacy Colleges
Aditya Nagar, ADB Road, Surampalem-533437 Kakinada District, Andhra Pradesh Ph: +91-9866576663, +91-9949876664
Email: office@acop.edu.in, office@adityapharmacy.edu.in

Editor: Dr. K. Ravishankar

ISBN: 9788197973123

ISBN: 9788197973123
Published by ThinkPlus Pharma Publications,
9-15/1, Indrapalem, Kakinada, AP-533006, India.
Website: www.books.jopir.in

Printed at Tarangini Printing Works, Subhadra Arcade, Bhanugudi, Kakinada, AP-533003, India.

DEDICATION

This conference proceedings are dedicated to Padma Bhushan Dr. K.I. Varaprasad Reddy garu, whose pioneering spirit and visionary leadership have revolutionized India's biotechnology landscape. His remarkable journey from an electronics engineer to a biotechnology pioneer, culminating in the development of India's first indigenous recombinant hepatitis B vaccine, serves as an inspiration to all. We honor his multidisciplinary expertise spanning defense science, industrial development, and biotechnology, as well as his commitment to making life-saving medications accessible to the common man. His generous sponsorship of this annual conference reflects his ongoing dedication to advancing scientific research and innovation in pharmaceutical sciences. His legacy of determination, innovation, and social responsibility continues to inspire the next generation of pharmaceutical scientists and researchers.

CONTENTS

ACKNOWLEDGMENTS

We express our profound gratitude to our publishing partners, the Journal of Clinical and Pharmaceutical Research and ThinkPlus® Pharma Publications, for their support in disseminating these proceedings. Special thanks to all the distinguished speakers, particularly Padma Bhushan Dr. K.I. Varaprasad Reddy, Dr. Montu M Patel, Dr. Anil Nilkanth Gaikwad, Dr. Chaganty Sreedhara, Prof. Dr. S Kavimani, Mr. K. Shyam Sundar, and Dr. M. Venkata Ramana for their valuable contributions. We acknowledge the tireless efforts of the organizing committee, faculty members, and staff of Aditya Group of Pharmacy Colleges in making this conference a success. Our appreciation extends to all participating researchers, academicians, and industry experts who shared their knowledge through paper presentations and discussions. We also thank the editorial board members for their meticulous review and guidance in maintaining the quality of these proceedings.

ACKNOWLEDGEMENTS

PREFACE

On behalf of the organizing committee of Aditya Group of Pharmacy Colleges, I am delighted to present the proceedings of the "Two-day National Conference on Computational Advancements in Research and Education for Pharmaceutical Excellence (CARE 2024)". This conference was held on 15th and 16th November 2024 at Surampalem to discuss the role of computational technologies in advancing research and education in the pharmaceutical sector.

The use of computational tools like artificial intelligence, machine learning, computer modeling and simulation is transforming various aspects of pharmaceutical research and education. These technologies are now playing a key role right from drug discovery and development to precision medicine and more. The conference aimed to bring together leading researchers, academics, industry experts and policymakers to explore emerging trends in areas like computational drug design, predictive toxicology, virtual clinical trials, personalized therapeutics and more. It also discussed strategies to integrate computational approaches better into pharmaceutical curricula and training programs. Over the two days, we had insightful paper presentations, case studies, panel discussions and interactive sessions that helped understand the impact and potential of computational technologies. This publication comprises the peer-reviewed full research papers presented at the conference. I thank all the authors for sharing their work and contributing to the growing knowledge base in this important domain.

I would also like to express my gratitude to our publishing partners, the Journal of Clinical and Pharmaceutical Research and ThinkPlus® Pharma Publications, for agreeing to publish these conference proceedings and disseminate the key discussions to a wider academic fraternity. I hope readers find this compilation insightful in charting the computational path to pharmaceutical excellence.

Dr. K. Ravishankar, *M.Pharm, Ph.D*
Organizing Director
Professor and Principal, Aditya College of Pharmacy

CHAIRMAN'S MESSAGE

I am pleased that the proceedings of the CARE 2024 national conference are published. This conference has successfully shed light on the role of computational technologies in advancing pharmaceutical research and education. I congratulate the organizing committee and thank all participants for their insightful contributions. Aditya Group of Institutions is committed to facilitating such knowledge sharing platforms and encouraging further development in this important area. The use of computational tools holds immense potential to address key challenges in drug discovery, personalized medicine and more. I am confident these proceedings will provide valuable insights and motivate wider adoption of computational approaches for pharmaceutical excellence.

Dr. N. Sesha Reddy, *M.A., B.L.*
Chairman, Aditya Group of Institutions

VICE CHAIRMAN'S MESSAGE

I am delighted to present this collection of research/review papers from CARE 2024 national conference. Computational technologies are transforming various domains within pharmaceutical sector and this conference has effectively elucidated their impact and potential. I appreciate the contributions from authors and publishing partners for archiving the key deliberations. This compilation will help broaden our knowledge of computational applications and guide continued progress in this area. My best wishes for more such insightful discussions and knowledge exchange in the future conferences. The innovative implementations of computational tools discussed here will undoubtedly accelerate pharmaceutical excellence in years to come.

Dr. N. Satish Reddy, *M.B.A, Ph.D*
Vice Chairman, Aditya Group of Institutions

SECRETARY'S MESSAGE

I congratulate the organizing committee for their diligent efforts that facilitated the timely release of CARE 2024 conference proceedings. As computational technologies increasingly permeate various facets of pharmaceutical sector, such discussion platforms assume greater importance. This compilation of research works deals with relevant issues and will serve as a valuable reference. On behalf of the Aditya Group of Institutions, I thank all stakeholders who supported in organizing this insightful knowledge exchange conference. Special commendations to authors, reviewers and publishing partners for documenting these discussions which aim to advance pharmaceutical excellence through computational innovation.

Sri. N. K. Deepak Reddy, *M.Tech*
Secretary, Aditya Group of Institutions

ORGANIZING SECRETARY MESSAGE

I take this opportunity to express my sincere gratitude to all eminent speakers, delegates and supporting partners who made CARE 2024 a resounding success. This conference achieved its objective of fostering enlightening dialogues on the role of computational technologies in pharmaceutical research and education. The publication of these conference proceedings is a timely initiative that will aid in disseminating the innovative works presented at the event. My heartfelt thanks to the authors, reviewers and journal partners for their invaluable contributions. As the Organizing Secretary, I am delighted that we could facilitate a platform for knowledge sharing through CARE 2024. I wish all the very best for future advancements through such forums focused on computational excellence in pharmaceutical sector.

Dr. D. Sathis Kumar, *M.Pharm, Ph.D*
Professor and Principal, Aditya Pharmacy College

PLENARY LECTURES

Speaker	Padmabushan Dr. K. I. VaraPrasad Reddy, Founder, Shantha Biotech

Topic: Utilizing Computational Tools to Accelerate Pharmaceutical Innovation

In his insightful keynote address at CARE 2024, Dr. K. I. VaraPrasad Reddy garu shared valuable insights from his experience leading India's biotech revolution with Shantha Biotech. Dr. Reddy reminisced about how technological disruptions like genetic engineering and fermentation aided Shantha in delivering cost-effective therapeutics.

He emphasized the need for the pharmaceutical industry to proactively adopt computational technologies like artificial intelligence, computer-aided molecular modeling and cloud-computing infrastructures to streamline R&D processes. Citing various real world examples, Dr. K. I. VaraPrasad Reddy garu underlined approaches to leverage computational drug design, predictive analytics and virtual clinical trials methodologies for accelerating research.

For transformation, he advocated collaborating with startups focused on healthcare informatics and establishing digitized and data-driven supply chains for informed decisions. Dr. Reddy concluded by encouraging the pharmaceutical sector to embrace computational advancements just as biotech leveraged opportune tools, to convert disruptions into opportunities and bolster excellence. Pioneering organizations like Shantha demonstrate a roadmap for computational-led pharmaceutical progress.

Speaker	Dr. Montu M Patel, President, Pharmacy Council of India

Topic: Computational Advancements for Quality Assurance and Regulation in Pharma Sector

As the head of the national pharmacy regulatory body, Dr. Patel shared PCI's perspective on leveraging computational tools for ensuring quality and compliance. He discussed ongoing initiatives employing technologies like AI, blockchain and virtual/augmented reality for drug quality monitoring and inspection processes.

Specific examples included AI-based real-time surveillance of supply chains, blockchain-driven serialization and e-audit trails. Dr. Patel also spoke about regulatory sandbox initiatives for novel digital therapeutics and personalized medicine tools.

He emphasized the need for collaborative efforts between regulatory agencies, academia and industry to establish digital infrastructure and harmonized standards. Dr. Patel encouraged partnerships to develop advanced in silico models for timely quality evaluations and protocol reviews through digital platforms. This can bolster patient safety and facilitate quicker access to quality therapies

Speaker	Dr. Anil Nilkanth Gaikwad, Sr. Pr. Scientist, Central Drug Research Institute, Lucknow

Topic: Next-Generation Computational Tools in Drug Metabolism Studies

Dr. Gaikwad delivered an enlightening presentation on revolutionary computational approaches transforming drug metabolism research. He demonstrated how advanced machine learning models are achieving unprecedented accuracy in predicting drug metabolism and toxicity profiles. The lecture highlighted their laboratory's groundbreaking work in quantum computing applications for modeling complex metabolic pathways and enzyme interactions. Through detailed case studies, he illustrated how their *in silico* methods successfully predicted drug-drug interactions and metabolite profiles with over 90% accuracy. Dr. Gaikwad emphasized that these computational tools can reduce animal testing requirements by up to 40% while accelerating drug development timelines significantly. He presented their novel hybrid approach combining artificial intelligence with traditional QSAR models for enhanced predictive power. The talk showcased recent developments in physiologically-based pharmacokinetic modeling and its seamless integration with AI platforms. Of particular interest was their work on deep learning algorithms for predicting rare metabolic reactions and identifying potential toxic metabolites early in drug development. Dr. Gaikwad concluded by presenting their upcoming projects on quantum-classical hybrid systems for real-time metabolism simulation and their potential impact on personalized medicine development.

Speaker	Dr. Chaganty Sreedhara, Principal Scientist III (ARD) Analaysis Lab Pvt Ltd

Topic: Analytical Excellence Through Computational Chemistry

Dr. Sreedhara presented a comprehensive overview of computational methods revolutionizing pharmaceutical analysis. He demonstrated their laboratory's pioneering work in implementing machine learning algorithms for complex spectral analysis and structural elucidation. The lecture showcased how their AI-powered analytical platform achieved a 60% reduction in analysis time while improving accuracy by 35%. He presented case studies of successful implementation in impurity profiling and stability testing, where neural networks automatically identified and quantified degradation products. Dr. Sreedhara explained their novel approach to computer-assisted method development, which optimizes analytical conditions using machine learning algorithms. A significant portion of the talk focused on their cloud-based analytical data management system, enabling real-time monitoring and analysis of multiple analytical instruments across different locations. He demonstrated their recent success in implementing natural language processing for automated analytical report generation and compliance documentation. The presentation included groundbreaking work on quantum computing applications in computational chemistry, particularly for modeling complex molecular structures. Dr. Sreedhara concluded by discussing future initiatives in developing AI-powered quality control systems and their potential impact on regulatory compliance.

Speaker	Prof Dr. S Kavimani, Principal and Professor, Mother Theresa PG and Research Institute

Topic: Digital Transformation in Pharmacy Education

Dr. Kavimani delivered an insightful presentation on revolutionizing pharmacy education through computational technologies. He showcased their institute's successful implementation of virtual laboratories and augmented reality platforms, which have significantly enhanced student understanding of complex pharmaceutical concepts. The lecture demonstrated their innovative AI-powered adaptive learning system, which personalizes educational content based on individual student performance and learning patterns. He presented compelling data showing a 40% improvement in student engagement and a 30% increase in practical skills acquisition through their digital learning platforms. Dr. Kavimani shared their experience in developing and implementing virtual manufacturing simulations, allowing students to practice GMP procedures and troubleshooting in a risk-free environment. The presentation highlighted their pioneering work in integrating computational drug design tools into the curriculum, preparing students for modern pharmaceutical research. He discussed their collaborative projects with industry partners to provide students with hands-on experience in using industry-standard computational tools. Dr. Kavimani emphasized their strategic approach to developing digital literacy and computational thinking skills among pharmacy students. The talk concluded with their roadmap for implementing emerging technologies like virtual reality and artificial intelligence in pharmacy education.

Speaker	Mr. K. Shyam Sundar, Technical Training Head-South Asia, USP NF

Topic: Quality Control Evolution Through Computational Methods

Mr. Sundar delivered a comprehensive presentation on USP's initiatives in modernizing quality control through computational approaches. He detailed their implementation of advanced machine learning algorithms for method validation and stability testing, which has reduced analysis time by 50% while improving reliability. The lecture showcased USP's innovative blockchain-based system for maintaining data integrity and traceability in pharmaceutical testing. He demonstrated their AI-powered platform for real-time monitoring of quality parameters and automated detection of out-of-specification results. The presentation included case studies of successful implementation of computational tools in various pharmacopeial procedures, showing significant improvements in accuracy and efficiency. Mr. Sundar highlighted USP's ongoing projects in developing standardized protocols for validating AI-based analytical methods. He presented their vision for integrating quantum computing in future quality control standards, particularly for complex molecular analysis. The talk addressed practical challenges in implementing computational methods in quality control laboratories and proposed solutions based on USP's global experience. Mr. Sundar concluded by outlining USP's upcoming initiatives in developing comprehensive guidelines for computational quality control methods.

Speaker	Dr. M. Venkata Ramana, Member of PCI Executive Committee

Topic: Regulatory Perspectives on Computational Pharmaceutical Sciences

Dr. Ramana presented a comprehensive overview of evolving regulatory frameworks for computational tools in pharmaceutical research and education. He detailed PCI's initiatives in developing guidelines for validating AI-based drug development methods and computational modeling tools. The lecture addressed critical challenges in regulating digital therapeutics and automated drug discovery platforms, emphasizing the need for balanced oversight. He presented case studies of successful regulatory approvals for computationally designed drugs and discussed lessons learned from these experiences. Dr. Ramana shared PCI's strategic plan for standardizing computational pharmacy curricula across India, including minimum computational competency requirements for pharmacy graduates. He highlighted their collaborative efforts with international regulatory bodies to harmonize standards for computational tools in drug development. The presentation included detailed discussions on data privacy considerations, validation requirements for AI models, and quality assurance protocols for computational methods. Dr. Ramana emphasized PCI's commitment to creating a regulatory environment that promotes innovation while ensuring patient safety. The talk concluded with upcoming regulatory changes designed to accommodate advanced computational methods while maintaining rigorous quality standards in pharmaceutical research and development

Ferroptosis In Cancer

Scan to View online

Presented by
Karrothu Akshaya, Allu Sirisha, Akshaya Karrothu, Durga Lakshmi Priya
Raghu College of Pharmacy,
Bheemunipatnam, Andhra Pradesh, India

Abstract

Apoptosis is a type of programmed cell death that differs from other forms such as autophagy and necroptosis. Ferroptosis, also a programmed cell death, occurs as a result of iron-dependent accumulation of lipid peroxides. It involves oxidative damage to the cell membrane by reactive oxygen species, resulting in cell death. This strategy is employed in treating various diseases like parkinson's and kidney damage. Different regulatory pathways, such as the gpx4 pathway, phospholipid metabolism pathway, iron metabolism pathway, and iron metabolism in mitochondria, mediate the process of ferroptosis. The agents that are responsible for the induction of ferroptosis in malignant cells are called ferroptosis inducers, such as small molecules and drugs, nucleic acids, and proteins(ASC, FSP, DHODH). Ferroptosis can be used in treating different cancers like glioblastoma, pancreatic cancer, breast cancer, head and neck, and also neurodegenerative diseases. Apolipoprotein e, involved in alzheimer's disease, can safely guard cells against several ferroptosis inducers, such as erastin. It prevents ferroptosis by decreasing iron release from ferritin through the akt pathway. There are different challenges in ferroptosis, such as biomarkers, selective targeting, drug resistance, heterogenicity.

Keywords: *Ferroptosis, ASC, FSP, DHODH, Glioblastoma cancer, ERASTIN cancer cells,*

Presented as Poster

A Novel Therapeutic Approach Of Targeted Nucleic Acid Delivery System

Scan to View online

Presented by
Teki Swathi Revathi Naga Lakshmi,
Sarampati Vishnu Surya Kala
Aditya Pharmacy College, Aditya University, Surampalem, Andhra Pradesh, India

Abstract

Nucleic acid delivery system is a technique designed for efficient delivery of nucleic acids (DNA, RNA) into cells to modify gene expression, treat genetic diseases or provide therapeutic benefits. Enhancement of gene therapy efficacy is done by developing targeted nanoparticles for nucleic acid delivery to view the advancements and challenges in gene therapy. Nucleic acids are the macromolecules which are used to carry information in cells, and also useful to makeup genetic material. Nucleic acid delivery systems are mainly based on two types of delivery systems they are, viral based delivery system and non-viral delivery system. Viral vectors mainly include retrovirus, adenovirus, adeno associated vectors. Non- viral delivery systems includes liposome delivery, nanoparticle delivery, electroporation, microinjection, gene gun. Gene therapy results in enhanced gene expression mechanism, targeted nanoparticles increased specificity, estimated delivery efficacy in invitro and invivo therapy system. Gene therapy is highly promising for clinical applications involving the insertion of a functioning nucleic acid into dysfunctioning cells to provide correct cellular function. Targeted nucleic acid delivery system holds potentiality for treating genetic diseases. Nucleic acid based therapeutic delivery system is the technique of gene therapy useful for treatment of many genetic disorders. This review highlights advancements and challenges, clinical and guiding researchers for more effective gene therapies.

Keywords: *Gene Therapy, Nucleic Acid Delivery, Precision Medicine, Targeted Delivery And Nanoparticles, Vector Based Delivery.*

Presented as Poster

A Break Through In Treating MDRTB - BPALM Regimen

Scan to View online

Presented by
Jain Jainam, B Surekha,K Swathi Tejasree,K Purna Nagasree
Raghu College of Pharmacy,
Bheemunipatnam, Andhra Pradesh, India

Abstract

Tuberculosis (TB) is an infectious disease that most often affects the lungs and is caused by a type of bacteria Mycobacterium tuberculosis. It spreads through the air when infected people cough, sneeze or spit. An estimated 10.6 million people effected with tuberculosis and 1.3 million people died from TB in 2023 as per WHO reports. India has incidence rate of 192 cases per 100,000 of population and in 2023, India accounted for 2.5million TB cases registered. Although there was treatment for TB like first line and second line drugs but their usage is for prolonged time and it is not assured that it can completely kill the tuberculosis bacteria. It stands for Bedaquiline, Pretomanid, Linezolid and Moxifloxacin. This combination therapy is part of newer treatments being developed to address multidrug resistant TB (MDR-TB) and extensively drug-resistant TB (XDR-TB). It has been a promising alternative due to shorter treatment durations and improved outcomes. The drugs were chosen because they target different critical bacterial functions— energy production, protein synthesis, cell wall synthesis, and DNA replication (targeting ATP synthase, DNA gyrase, Topoisomerase IV) -providing a robust and multi-pronged attack on Mycobacterium tuberculosis. This new treatment duration is very short that is 6 months as compared to older therapy of 18-24 months. This therapy is approved by CDSCO in India on 06/10/2024 and approved by US FDA on 09/05/2023.

Keywords: *Tuberculosis,MDR-TB,BPaLM,Bedaquiline ,pretomanid*

Presented as Poster

Advances In CRISPR-Based Organoid Models For Studying Hereditary Kidney Diseases

Scan to View online

Presented by
Sara Aiswarya Bommeti, Dr. Praveen Sana.
Aditya Pharmacy College, Aditya University, Surampalem, Andhra Pradesh, India

Abstract

Gene technology, CRISPR-CAS9(clustered regularly interspaced short palindromic repeats- CRISPR-associated protein 9), is always challenging as it represents a revolutionary approach toward the treatment of hereditary kidney diseases, autosomal dominant polycystic kidney disease, and alport syndrome. This technology can change the dna sequence of the genetic mutation; therefore, it significantly advances curative treatments in a patient suffering from hereditary kidney disease. These experimental techniques on animal models of these diseases performed well in suppressing cyst formation, fibrosis, and proteinuria of the kidneys. However, difficulties remain regarding the specific delivery of the crispr components to the kidney tissue. Nanoparticles and viral vectors are some of the more complex delivery systems studied with tighter targeting specificity and a reduced off-target effect. Several issues regarding efficiency, safety, and specific ethical implications will have to be solved before crispr can be put in place on a wide scale at the level of ethical and safety issues as well as long-term clinical implications. More studies will be needed before the technical as well as ethical challenges are resolved to allow crispr to find its place in nephrology on a wide scale. However, the crispr potential is transformative and may soon be realized shortly when personalized curative therapies for genetic kidney disorders start to increasingly feature in medical treatments.

Keywords: *CRISPR-CAS9, Alport Syndrome, Nanoparticles, Polycystic Kidney Disease, Hereditary Kidney Disease, Fibrosis.*

Presented as Poster

Magneto-Pharmacology An Emerging Trend

Scan to View online

Presented by
M.Sivamani, Nikhil .J
Aditya Pharmacy College, Aditya University, Surampalem, Andhra Pradesh, India

Abstract

Magneto-pharmacology is an emerging area that combines magnetic systems with active pharmaceutical ingredients to adjust drug delivery. The usage of magnetic materials to manipulate and direct drug carriers which include nanoparticles pursuits to amelioration the targeting and efficacy of medical treatments even as decreasing side effects. The development of superparamagnetic nanoparticles is paving the manner for particular targeting of medication to tissues, such as tumors, enhancing the remedy of illnesses along with cancer and neurological diseases. Antimagnetic tablets that enable managed launch from external magnetic fields had been added. This potential allows for adjustment of dosage and length, which is essential for persistent illnesses that require lengthy-term treatment. In addition, the mixing of imaging era with magnetic medicinal drug makes it beneficial for monitoring drug distribution and remedy efficacy. I'm nevertheless there. However, the capacity applications of magneto-pharmacology in precision medicinal drug are large and provide new thoughts to conquer the limitations of conventional treatment options. Through collaborative collaboration, magnet pharmacology has the ability to revolutionize scientific practice and facilitate the development of targeted remedies.

Keywords: *Magneto-Pharmacology, Superparamagnetic, Nanoparticles, Persistent Illness, Neurological.*

Presented as Poster

Brain Chip Technology

Scan to View online

Presented by
D.Swathi, A.B.T.M.Lakshmi, G.K.Goutami, G.Nitya Sri
Sri Vasavi Institute of Pharmaceutical Sciences, Pedatadepalli, Andhra Pradesh, India

Abstract

Brain chip technology or brain computer interface (BCI)enables direct communication between the brain and external devices.Elon Musk and his team members contribute great efforts in its development.Different types of brain chip implants are available,some of them directly implanted into brain tissue and some of them are implanted into skull but not brain tissue .It is a computer based system that acquires brain signals,analyses them and translates them in to commands that are connected to an output device to carry out the desired action. Although it has some drawbacks such as High cost ,rejection of implants and hacking of brain they have significant advantages such as enhancing memory of humans and give paralysed patients full mental control on limbs and for military purposes such as testing of soldier cognitive work load,and useful to treat to neural disorders. It also give hope to partially or fully blind patients in the form of bionic eye . Bionic eye is the one of example of brain chip technology in which chip is implanted in visual cortex of brain helps to restore the eye functions

Keywords: *Brain chip, Bionic eye, cognitive enhancement, Neural implant, Neural disorders*

Presented as Poster

Key Developments And Emerging Trends In Neuropsychological Assessment

Scan to View online

Presented by
Sri Harshitha Manchala, Rajeswari Makireddy, Parinaya Sri
Aditya Pharmacy College, Aditya University, Surampalem, Andhra Pradesh, India

Abstract

Neuropsychological assessment tools play a critical role in understanding the relationship between brain function and behavior. Over the past 40–50 years, the creation of standardized tests sensitive to these relationships has shaped how we approach questions about brain function, detect neurological disorders, and guide treatment. This review outlines key milestones and innovations in neuropsychological assessment, focusing on the evolution of tools used in current practice. Additionally, we highlight emerging research aimed at improving diagnostic and treatment outcomes by deepening our understanding of brain function. We provide a brief historical overview of major assessment approaches, including the lurian method, flexible and fixed batteries, and the boston process approach. We also discuss critical advancements in areas such as the use of normative standards, accounting for cultural differences, tracking longitudinal changes, and developing common metric batteries. Furthermore, we explore new trends in the field, including technological innovations, the integration of neuropsychology into other disciplines like primary care, and shifts in the assessment infrastructure. While neuropsychological assessment has grown significantly in recent decades, many challenges remain in improving measurement tools and translating findings into meaningful clinical recommendations.

Keywords: *Psychometrics, Cognitive Testing, Cross-Cultural, Computerized Assessment, Normative Standards*

Presented as Poster

Rheumatoid Arthritis

Scan to View online

Presented by
Sunadh, Chandu , Srinivas , Manikanta
Adarsa College Of Pharmacy,
G.Kothapalli, Andhra Pradesh, India

Abstract

Rheumatoid arthritis (ra) is a chronic, autoimmune inflammatory disorder that primarily affects the synovial joints, leading to pain, swelling, stiffness, and progressive joint destruction. It can also have systemic manifestations involving the lungs, heart, eyes, and blood vessels. The exact etiology remains unclear, but genetic predisposition, environmental factors, and immune dysregulation play significant roles in its development. Ra predominantly affects women and often manifests between the ages of 30 and 60. Diagnosis is based on clinical symptoms, blood tests for markers such as rheumatoid factor (rf) and anti-cyclic citrullinated peptide (anti-ccp) antibodies, and imaging studies. Early intervention is crucial to prevent irreversible joint damage. Treatment includes disease-modifying antirheumatic drugs (dmards), biologic agents, non-steroidal anti-inflammatory drugs (nsaids), corticosteroids, and lifestyle modifications. A multidisciplinary approach involving rheumatologists, physical therapists, and mental health professionals is essential for optimal disease management. Advances in treatment strategies have improved long-term outcomes, although challenges remain in achieving sustained remission and managing comorbidities.

Keywords: *Rheumatoid arthritis (RA) Autoimmune disorder Chronic inflammation Synovial joints Joint pain Rheumatoid factor (RF)*

Presented as Poster

Quality Control Of Ayurvedic Proprietary Medicine In Oral Health Care

Scan to View online

Presented by
Dhwani Patel
Parul Institute of Pharmacy and Research, Parul University, Waghodia, Gujarat, India

Abstract

Ayurveda, an ancient Indian traditional system of medicine that outlines treatment approaches and medicines based on herbs and their parts which offers a holistic approach to health and wellness, including oral care. Dental caries, periodontal diseases, gingivitis, are commonly occurring oral health problems. It is the one of the major issue of concern as the oral cavity is the window into the overall health of patient. Ayurveda practices use of dantdhavan, mouth wash, tooth-powder, oil-pulling, and gandoosha. Plants and derived products offers rich source of biologically active phytoconstituents. The increasing demand for ayurvedic products, concerns about quality control, safety and efficiency. To overcome this concern of matter, standardization and quality control testing of raw material used is important to guarantee their safety & efficiency. Quality control is a systemic approach that involves monitoring & controlling various aspects of herbal product. Also, one of the major aspect of quality control is assay of phytoconstitutent having therapeutic effect and also ensuring the consistency of quality in the rm which may differ due to different origin and nature. It is crucial to employ authentic methods in quality control of ayurvedic medication products to accurately identify herb which ensures that correct herb is utilized for specific oral problem. This topic aims to compile quality control parameters for the testing and maintaining quality of the ayurvedic products for oral healthcare

Keywords: *Quality control , phytoconstitutent, dental caries , raw material , standardization, ayurvedic products*

Presented as Poster

Implementation Of National Education Policy In Pharmacy Education

Scan to View online

Presented by
Sirapurapu Manjula
Aditya Pharmacy College, Aditya University, Surampalem, Andhra Pradesh, India

Abstract

The national education policy focusing on transforming india's education system, views on practical skills and real-world application.the goal is to give professionals who can innovate, research, and provide quality healthcare. To achieve this, pharmacy education is undergoing many changes.pharmacy students will now learn multidisciplinary sciences like chemistry, physics and biology in addition to pharmacy. This will help them understand the bigger picture and work accurately with other healthcare professionals. Partnerships with pharmaceutical companies will provide hands-on experience, preparing students for the industry. Teachers are being trained to choose to take modern teaching methods, emphasizing critical thinking and problem-solving skills. This will enable students to adapt to the ever-evolving healthcare landscape.there are numerous benefits for pharmacists.they will have best job prospects, both in india and internationally. Entrepreneurship will flourish, with pharmacists starting their own businesses and creating innovative solutions.however, challenges persist. Addressing these challenges needs collaboration between educators, policymakers, and industry leaders.by performing these changes, India can produce pharmacists who make a drastic change in healthcare. The national education policy's vision for pharmacy education is clear: to create professional convert healthcare and improve lives.

Keywords: *National Education Policy,Pharmacy Education,Interdisciplinary Learning,Practical Skills,healthcare Innovation*

Presented as Poster

A Breakthrough In Treating MDR TB-Bpalm Regimen

Scan to View online

Presented by
Jain Jainam, B.Surekha, K.Swathi Teja Sree,K.Purna Nagasree
Raghu College of Pharmacy,
Bheemunipatnam, Andhra Pradesh, India

Abstract

Tuberculosis (TB) is an infectious disease that most often affects the lungs and is caused by a type of bacteria Mycobacterium tuberculosis. It spreads through the air when infected people cough, sneeze or spit. An estimated 10.6 million people effected with tuberculosis and 1.3 million people died from TB in 2023 as per WHO reports. India has incidence rate of 192 cases per 100,000 of population and in 2023, India accounted for 2.5million TB cases registered. Although there was treatment for TB like first line and second line drugs but their usage is for prolonged time and it is not assured that it can completely kill the tuberculosis bacteria. Due to that the novel drug treatment was introduced that is called as BPaLM therapy. It stands for Bedaquiline, Pretomanid, Linezolid and Moxifloxacin. This combination therapy is part of newer treatments being developed to address multidrug resistant TB (MDR-TB) and extensively drug-resistant TB (XDR-TB). The drugs were chosen because they target different critical bacterial functions— energy production, protein synthesis, cell wall synthesis, and DNA replication (targeting ATP synthase, DNA gyrase, Topoisomerase IV) -providing a robust and multi-pronged attack on Mycobacterium tuberculosis. This new treatment duration is very short that is 6 months as compared to older therapy of 18-24 months. This therapy is approved by CDSCO in India on 06/10/2024 and approved by US FDA on 09/05/2023.

Keywords: *Tuberculosis, MDR-TB, BPaLM regimen, Bedaquiline,Pretomanid, Linezolid, Moxifloxacin*

Presented as Poster

New Computational Approaches On Anti Cancer Drug Discovery

Scan to View online

Presented by
A.S.N.S.S.L.Srividya , G.Tejaswi ,
K.P.B.Satvika , K.Naga Komali .
Sri Vasavi Institute of Pharmaceutical Sciences, Pedatadepalli, Andhra Pradesh, India

Abstract

Malignancies are a major health issue that account for one out of every six deaths worldwide. Aside from significant advancements in immunotherapies, stem cell transplantation, targeted therapies, hormone therapies, precision medicine, palliative care, and conventional medicines like chemotherapy, radiation therapy, and surgery, cancer therapy has always been difficult. Natural products give the scientific community the chance to investigate new natural compounds against tumors and are essential to the development of novel anticancer medications in cancer research. Using betulinic acid and withaferin A as examples, *in-vitro* and *in vivo* investigations have demonstrated the shift from computational to experimental validation. The difficulties and restrictions in creating natural compounds as possible anticancer medications are also covered . Furthermore, the anticancer potential of natural products may be improved by combining deep learning and artificial intelligence with conventional computational drug discovery techniques.

Keywords: *Malignancy ,Natural products, Medicine, Artifical intelligence ,Therapies*

Presented as Poster

Challenges Of Pcod Women And Future Aspects On Infertility Condition

Scan to View online

Presented by
P. Sai Priyanka, S. Hema Sri, N. Keerthi, P. Sailaja
VJ's College of Pharmacy, Rajahmundry, Andhra Pradesh, India

Abstract

Polycystic Ovary Syndrome (PCOS) is a common hormonal disorder that affects many women of reproductive age. It can cause various issues, including irregular menstrual cycles and difficulties with ovulation, which may lead to infertility. This can be particularly distressing for those trying to conceive. While there is no cure for PCOS, effective management is crucial. This includes adopting a healthy lifestyle with a balanced diet low in refined sugars, regular exercise, and stress management. Medical treatments such as birth control pills can help regulate periods, and medications like metformin can improve insulin sensitivity. For women trying to get pregnant, doctors may prescribe medications to help induce ovulation. With proper management, many women with PCOS can have healthy pregnancies. It's important to have regular check-ups to monitor any potential risks, such as gestational diabetes and high blood pressure. Maintaining a healthy lifestyle continues to support both the mother and the baby. By working closely with healthcare providers, women with PCOS can navigate their symptoms and enjoy a successful pregnancy journey.

Keywords: *PCOS, Endocrine disorder, Sensitizers, Ovulation induction, Pregnancy, Gestational diabetes, Healthcare providers.*

Presented as Poster

Method Development And Validation For The Simultaneous Estimation Of Allopurinol And Lisenurad Using HPLC

Scan to View online

Presented by
Kruthiventi Sai Priyanka,Sree Gayatri Aditya College of Pharmacy, Aditya University, Surampalem, Andhra Pradesh, India

Abstract

A simple, accurate, precise method was developed for the simultaneous estimation of allopurinol and lesinurad in tablet dosage form using rp-hplc method. Chromatogram was run through xterra c18 (4.6*150mm, 5μ) column. Mobile phase containing 0.1% OPA and methanol taken in the ratio of 60: 40 was pumped through column at a flow rate of 1ml/min. Temperature was maintained at ambient temperature. Optimized wavelength for both drugs was 255nm. Retention time of allopurinol and lesinurad were found to be 2.252min and 3.009min. % assay was obtained as 99.98% and 99.61% for allopurinol and lesinurad respectively. The linearity range was found to lie from 30μg/ml to 150μg/ml of allopurinol, 20μg/ml to 100μg/ml of lesinurad. It was concluded that our method consume less mobile phase with short running time with good resolution. So our developed method was simple and economical that can be adopted in regular quality control test in industries

Keywords: *Allopurinol, Lesinurad, RP-HPLC, Linearity, Precision*

Presented as Poster

Artificial Intelligence In Pharmacy Successful Pharmacological Discovery

Scan to View online

Presented by
A.Jyothi, P.Navyasri
VJ's College of Pharmacy, Rajahmundry, Andhra Pradesh, India

Abstract

Artificial Intelligence (AI) is revolutionizing the field of drug discovery by significantly accelerating the traditionally lengthy and costly process of bringing new therapeutics to market. By leveraging advanced computational techniques such as machine learning, deep learning, and natural language processing, AI enables researchers to identify drug candidates, optimize compounds, and predict drug-target interactions with unprecedented efficiency. AI facilitates multiple stages of drug discovery, including target identification, lead compound screening, and optimization, as well as drug repurposing and personalized medicine. Key successes, such as Insilico Medicine's AI-designed drug candidate for idiopathic pulmonary fibrosis (IPF)and DeepMind's AlphaFold for protein structure prediction, illustrate AI's transformative potential. These tools help reduce development costs, increase the probability of success, and expedite the time to clinical trials. Despite the immense promise, challenges remain regarding data quality, model interpretability, and regulatory hurdles. Continued advancements in AI methodologies, coupled with collaborations between academia, industry, and regulatory bodies, are expected to drive further innovations, leading to more effective, targeted, and safer therapeutics. AI's role in drug discovery heralds a new era of precision medicine, promising to address unmet medical needs and improve patient outcomes globa

Keywords: *Drug Repurposing: Real-World Examples, Drug development*

Presented as Poster

Redifining Diagnostics : The Rise Of Wireless Capsule Endoscopy In Modern Medicine

Scan to View online

Presented by
Nikhitha Mantena
Srinivasa Rao College of Pharmacy,
Visakhapatnam, Andhra Pradesh, India

Abstract

Wireless capsule endoscopy (WCE) has transformed gastrointestinal diagnostics by offering a non-invasive approach to examine the digestive system without the need for sedation or the risks of conventional endoscopic procedures. With proven effectiveness in detecting gastrointestinal tissue irregularities, particularly within the small intestine, WCE continues to gain importance. However, current commercial WCE devices have limitations, primarily due to their lack of autonomous lesion detection and treatment capabilities. Recent advancements in micro-electromechanical systems (MEMS) and computational technologies have driven intensive research focused on integrating sophisticated functionalities into WCE devices, with the ultimate aim of creating intelligent capsule robots that could surpass traditional wired endoscopes. By analyzing the potential benefits and drawbacks of these approaches, we highlight the emerging capabilities that could transform WCE devices into autonomous "capsule surgeons." These innovations foreshadow a future where capsule robots self-navigate and perform minimally invasive interventions within the gastrointestinal tract, suggesting a paradigm shift that may ultimately reduce or eliminate the need for direct physician involvement. The anticipated advancements in WCE promise a minimally invasive future in GI diagnostics and treatment, setting a new standard in non-invasive medical technology.

Keywords: *Wireless capsule endoscopy, Non-invasive diagnostics, Gastrointestinal Imaging, Intelligent capsule robots*

Presented as Poster

Multimodal Biomedical Ai: The Frontier In Pharmaceutical Innovation

Scan to View online

Presented by
E.Prasanna
School of Pharmaceutical Sciences & Technologies, JNTU, Kakinada, Andhra Pradesh, India

Abstract

The integration of artificial intelligence (AI) in healthcare has transformed pharmaceutical research and personalized medicine. Traditional methods often face limitations due to fragmented data analysis, reducing their effectiveness in tackling complex diseases. Multimodal Biomedical AI, which merges data from genomics, medical imaging, and electronic health records (EHR), offers a breakthrough by providing a unified approach to solving these challenges. Platforms like IBM Watson and Google's DeepMind applied multimodal AI to analyze large-scale clinical data, recommend treatments, and predict patient outcomes, expediting vaccine development and therapeutic discoveries.In cancer treatment, genomic sequencing identifies mutations and genetic markers that influence tumor behavior. Deep learning models such as Convolutional Neural Networks (CNNs) for imaging and Natural Language Processing (NLP) for analyzing clinical data synthesize these insights, enabling precision therapies tailored to the patient's genetic profile. This technology optimizes drug discovery, improves patient selection in clinical trials, and enhances pharmacovigilance by predicting drug responses and adverse reactions. With its success during COVID-19, multimodal AI is advancing cancer treatments and ensuring more personalized therapies.

Keywords: *Multimodal Biomedical AI, Multi omics, Deep learning, Convolutional Neural Networks4, Natural Language Processing5..*

Presented as Poster

Comparison Of Fixed And Variable Loop Button Fixation In Arthroscopic Anterior Cruciate Ligament Reconstruction

Scan to View online

Presented by
B.Mounika, R.Priyanka, A.Lokesh,
Dr.Surya Prakash Naidu
Aditya Pharmacy College, Aditya University, Surampalem, Andhra Pradesh, India

Abstract

A maximum number of grafts can be positioned inside the femoral tunnel thanks to the development of fixed- and variable-loop suspensory fixation devices for arthroscopic anterior cruciate ligament (ACL) restoration. Few comparative clinical studies exist despite several biomechanical investigations comparing these two devices. This study aimed to compare the functional outcomes of arthroscopic acl reconstruction utilizing fixed-loop devices with those of variable-loop devices by examining their impact on graft laxity clinical assessment and patient-reported outcome scores. In acl reconstruction, the fixation of grafts within the femoral tunnel is critical to achieving optimal graft tension, stability, and long-term durability. Fixed-loop devices have a set loop length, providing a more rigid fixation. In contrast, variable-loop devices allow for adjustable loop lengths, potentially offering better control over graft tension and positioning. A typical surgical technique for regaining knee stability and function is anterior cruciate ligament (acl) reconstruction. Suspensory fixation tools, especially fixed- and variable-loop buttons, are essential for femoral tunnel graft fixation and have an effect on the results of surgery. Clinical evidence comparing the functional outcomes of the devices is few, despite biomechanical studies suggesting that each device offers unique advantages in graft stability.

Keywords: *Anterior Cruciate Ligament (ACL) reconstruction ,Suspensory Fixation Devices, Fixed-Loop Devices, Variable-Loop Devices ,Femoral Tunnel*

Presented as Poster

Computational Advancements In Pharmacogenomics: The Future Of Personalized Medicine

Scan to View online

Presented by
Amana Mohammed Ahmad, Yerra Sharmila, Kona Krishna Sri
School of Pharmaceutical Sciences & Technologies, JNTU, Kakinada, Andhra Pradesh, India

Abstract

Pharmacogenomics, the study of how genes affect a person's response to drugs, has experienced significant computational advancements in recent years, revolutionizing personalized medicine. Integrating large-scale genomic data with computational tools has enabled researchers to identify genetic variations that influence drug metabolism, efficacy, and safety. High-throughput sequencing technologies, coupled with advanced bioinformatics algorithms, facilitate the analysis of vast datasets, allowing for the discovery of novel pharmacogenomic markers. Machine learning and artificial intelligence are increasingly employed to predict patient responses to medications based on genetic profiles, enhancing the ability to tailor treatments to individual patients. These computational methods also streamline the drug development process by identifying patient populations likely to benefit from specific therapies, thus optimizing clinical trial designs and improving success rates. Additionally, the use of computational models to simulate drug interactions at the molecular level aids in understanding complex biological pathways, further informing therapeutic strategies. As electronic health records (EHRs) increasingly incorporate genomic information, computational tools can provide real-time insights into patient care, promoting the implementation of pharmacogenomic data in clinical settings.

Keywords: *Pharmacogenomics, Personalized medicine, Computational models, Machine learning , Key tools, Electronic Health Records*

Presented as Poster

Bilosomes In Novel Drug Delivery System

Scan to View online

Presented by
Vijaya Lakshmi, Raga Surekha, Lakshmi Surekha
Aditya College of Pharmacy, Aditya University, Surampalem, Andhra Pradesh, India

Abstract

Bilosomes are novel, bile salt-based vesicular carriers primarily used for oral drug delivery systems. These nanocarriers are formed by incorporating bile salts into liposomes, which enhances their stability and bioavailability, especially in the harsh conditions of the gastrointestinal (gi) tract. Due to the presence of bile salts, bilosomes exhibit resistance to bile acid-induced degradation, allowing them to improve drug absorption and protect encapsulated bioactive agents, including vaccines, proteins, and peptides. This feature makes them suitable for non-invasive delivery of therapeutics that would otherwise be degraded in the GI tract, presenting a promising strategy for enhancing the oral bioavailability of various drugs and biologics.

Keywords: *Bilosomes, Drug Delivery system, Oral vaccines*

Presented as Poster

Mouth Dissolving Tablets

Scan to View online

Presented by
N.Kamakshi,K.Naveena , N.Bannu
Raghu College of Pharmacy,
Bheemunipatnam, Andhra Pradesh, India

Abstract

Mouth-dissolving tablets (MDTs), also known as orally disintegrating tablets (ODTs), are a type of fast-dissolving medication designed to dissolve or disintegrate quickly in the mouth without the need for water. Developed to improve patient compliance and ease of administration, especially for populations with swallowing difficulties (like pediatric and geriatric patients), MDTs utilize specialized formulations that allow for rapid breakdown upon contact with saliva. This rapid dissolution ensures a faster onset of action compared to traditional tablets, making them suitable for medications requiring prompt therapeutic effects, such as analgesics or antihistamines. MDTs are prepared through various methods, including freeze-drying, spray drying, and direct compression.Emerging innovations continue to refine the formulation and production of MDTs, making them a growing sector within pharmaceutical development aimed at enhancing patient experience and compliance across various therapeutic areas.

Keywords: *Disintegrants, Dissolvents , Mouth Dissolving Tablets,*

Presented as Poster

Artificial Intelligence In Clinical Trails At Present Scenario

Scan to View online

Presented by
P.Sri Sai Mounika Reddy, P.Jahnavi, M.Ramya Sri, K.Jahnavi Sravanthi
Lydia College of Pharmacy, Ethakota, Ravulapalem, Andhra Pradesh, India

Abstract

Delivering new drugs, technologies, and procedures to the market and practice requires clinical trails. Due to the increasing cost and complexity of conducting clinical trails, only 10% of these studies finish the entire process, from drug design to the four stages of development. This low completion rate had a significant negative impact on the population's sustainability, standard treatment, health economics, and health. One of the tools that could expedite some of the most laborious procedures, such as patient selection, matching and enrollment, is artificial intelligence(AI); better patient selection could also reduce harmful treatment and its side effects. There are still many obstacles in the way of the wide spread use of AI technology in clinical trails, and more high-caliber prospective clinical validation is needed.

Keywords: *Laborious, Sustainability, Health economics,clinical validation,obstacles*

Presented as Poster

Investigation Of Keratolytic Activity Using Azadiracta Indica Ointment Preparataion.

Scan to View online

Presented by
D. Jayasri, D. Vijaya Lakshmi, G. Raga Surekha, G. Mahitha, G. Aishwarya.
Aditya College of Pharmacy, Aditya University, Surampalem, Andhra Pradesh, India

Abstract

Skin issues are very common, and keratosis is one of the skin conditions which gets worse in the winter season effecting people with eczema, sometimes dermatitis leading to open heeled or broken heels resulting in inflammation and pain. The best natural skin care selected for the current study to treat keratosis is by preparing an indigenous semi-solid dosage form using azadiracta indica extract as active ingredient. 10% azadiracta indica extract is incorporated with various ingredients like hard paraffin, cetosteryl alcohol, wool fat, white soft paraffin and little quantity of glycerin. The ointment is applied to the affected areas twice daily for a period of 3 to 7 days. There is a marked improvement, and this formulation is found to possess excellent keratolytic activity. The formulated ointment activity is compared with standard 5% salicylic acid ointment.

Keywords: *Azadiracta Indica, Keratosis, Salicylic Acid, Formulation, Eczema, Dermatitis.*

Presented as Poster

Menstrual Disorders

Scan to View online

Presented by
Venkata Lakshmi, Gayatri, Akhila,
Sravanthi
Adarsa College Of Pharmacy,
G.Kothapalli, Andhra Pradesh, India

Abstract

Menstrual disorders encompass a range of conditions that affect the normal menstrual cycle, leading to variations in frequency, regularity, duration, and intensity of menstrual bleeding. Common menstrual disorders include amenorrhea (absence of menstruation), dysmenorrhea (painful periods), menorrhagia (heavy menstrual bleeding), oligomenorrhea (infrequent periods), and premenstrual syndrome (pms). These disorders can be caused by hormonal imbalances, structural abnormalities, underlying medical conditions, lifestyle factors, or stress. They often impact women's physical and emotional well-being, productivity, and quality of life. Diagnosis involves a combination of medical history, physical examination, blood tests, and imaging techniques. Treatment strategies range from lifestyle modifications and pharmacological interventions—such as hormonal therapies, pain management, and non-steroidal anti-inflammatory drugs (nsaids)—to surgical options in severe cases. A multidisciplinary approach involving gynecologists, endocrinologists, and mental health professionals is often necessary for effective management

Keywords: *Menstrual disorders Amenorrhea Dysmenorrhea Menorrhagia Oligomenorrhea Polymenorrhea*

Presented as Poster

Emerging Therapies In Chronic Kidney Disease: Advancements In Cardiovascular Risk Management And Renal Protection

Scan to View online

Presented by
Lalitha Maheswari Dandipati, Dr. D. V. S. Somayajulu, Himabindu Gudimetla, Pushpa Satya Mahalakshmi Sanivarapu
Aditya Pharmacy College, Aditya University, Surampalem, Andhra Pradesh, India

Abstract

It has become increasingly evident that the treatment of chronic kidney disease (ckd), along with its spectrum of high cardiovascular risk in the general population across the world, encompasses new therapies such as angiotensin receptor/neprilysin inhibitors, sodium glucose transporter 2 inhibitors, glucagon-like peptide-1 receptor agonists, and finerenone. Extensive literature searches identified the ckd treatments emerging: SGLT2 inhibitors, arni, glp-1 agonists, and finerenone. Non-english studies, case reports, and small trials with non-important outcomes were excluded. The methodologies of the studies selected, populations, interventions, and outcomes were reviewed. The primary therapeutic options encompass arni and SGLT2 inhibitors, both of which demonstrate a significant advantage in reducing cardiovascular and renal outcomes in individuals with ckd. Furthermore, arni offers additional cardiovascular protection in the context of heart failure, while sglt2 inhibitors confer a multifaceted benefit, potentially influencing glucose regulation alongside renal safeguarding. Patients exhibiting nephrotic range proteinuria alongside inadequately managed blood pressure represent a demographic that has not been extensively researched. It is essential to address the unique challenges faced by these groups in the context of chronic kidney disease (CKD) management.

Keywords: *Finerenone, Neprilysin Inhibitors, SGLT2 Inhibitors, Arni, GLP-1 Receptor Agonists, Hyperkalaemia.*

Presented as Poster

Preliminary Phytochemical Screening And Anti-Anemic Activity Of Crotalaria Juncea Whole Plant Extract

Scan to View online

Presented by
L Siddu, M. Ravi Syamala, M.Kiran Kumar, M.D. Saahul, M. Swapna.
Aditya College of Pharmacy, Aditya University, Surampalem, Andhra Pradesh, India

Abstract

Crotalaria juncea familiar as sun hemp, abundantly available in many parts of andhra pradesh and the plant is being used by local natives as a medicine for the treatment of pain and skin diseases. The whole plant extract was evaluated for anti-anemic activity. The standard agent phenyl hydrazine is injected to albino rats and notable decline in hemoglobin levels and red blood cell count is noted in experimental albino rats. The crotalaria juncea extract at a dose of 200 and 400 mg/kg when given to albino rats there is a marked exalted levels of hemoglobin and red blood cell count to an appreciable extent. Further, these parameters were compared with standard hematinic agent ferrous ascorbate.

Keywords: *Crotalaria Juncea, Phenyl Hydrazine, Ferrous Ascorbate, Anemia, Red Blood Cells, Hemoglobin.*

Presented as Poster

Computational Technologies In Management Of Oncology

Scan to View online

Presented by
Keerthi, Kiranmai, Greeshma Durga , Pavani
Viswanadha Institute of Pharmaceutical Sciences, Sontyam, Visakhapatnam, Andhra Pradesh, India

Abstract

Computational technologies are playing a pivotal role in advancing oncology by enabling more precise, personalized, and effective cancer treatments. This topic discusses the integration of four key technologies—genome editing, immunotherapy, artificial intelligence (AI), and nanotechnology—that are transforming the landscape of cancer research and care. The technology allows precise alterations in the DNA of cancer cells , enabling researches to target specific genes responsible for cancer development resistance and metastasis. It uses computational models to optimize immune response, has gained prominence with advancements like CAR-T cell therapy, which harnesses the immune system to recognize and destroy cancer cells. Powered algorithms are significantly enhancing early detection, personalized treatment plans, and predictive outcomes by analyzing large-scale clinical and genomic data. It contributes to oncology by improving drug delivery mechanisms, allowing for precision-targeted therapies that minimize damage to healthy tissues and reduce side effects. The integration of these computational technologies is ushering in a new era of cancer treatment, where therapies are more efficient, targeted, and tailored to the individual patient's genetic and molecular profile. This abstract provides insights into current applications, challenges, and future prospects of these technologies in revolutionizing oncology care.

Keywords: *Genome editing, CRISPR-cas9, immunotherapy, CAR-T, AI,Nanotechnology*

Presented as Poster

Dominance Of Fruquintinib: Recent Booming Of Metastatic Colorectal Cancer Treatment

Scan to View online

Presented by
M. Sujith, Sk. Meerjavalli
VJ's College of Pharmacy, Rajahmundry, Andhra Pradesh, India

Abstract

The recent concern about the colorectal cancer is exponentially increasing due to the major risk factors are being considerable for its ranking of3rddangerous contingency and 4th leading one in cancer deaths over the eastern Asia. The US FDA approved drug for this major metastatic cancer is fruquintinib (Fruzaqla, Takeda Pharmaceuticals, Inc.); it is potent, TKI, and orally active in nature. This approval was granted on 8th November 2023 based on selectivity of VEGFR-1,2,3 tyrosine kinases inhibition as the differentiating factor and dominant in nature among other therapies. There are several treatments for mCRC this above drug falls into the category of targeted therapy. There have been 75 clinical trials gone so far in which the most recent clinical trial was a phase 3 trial, which was initiated on 1st January 2023 that responded in a positive rate of 95% of success rate and having disease control rate [DCR] of 56% that is notable.This explains that patients treated with fruquintinib had a significantly higher objective response compared to placebo.

Keywords: *Colorectal cancer Fruquintinib VEGFR kinases Targeted cancer therapy*

Presented as Poster

Thyroid Disorder

Scan to View online

Presented by
Joshna, Ratnam, Madhuri
Adarsa College Of Pharmacy,
G.Kothapalli, Andhra Pradesh, India

Abstract

Thyroid disorders are a group of conditions affecting the structure or function of the thyroid gland, leading to disruptions in hormone production and metabolic regulation. The most common disorders include hypothyroidism (underactive thyroid), hyperthyroidism (overactive thyroid), thyroiditis (inflammation of the thyroid), and goiter (enlarged thyroid), as well as autoimmune conditions such as hashimoto's thyroiditis and graves' disease. Thyroid dysfunction can result from genetic predisposition, iodine deficiency, autoimmune responses, or environmental factors. Symptoms vary based on the type of disorder and may include fatigue, weight changes, mood disturbances, cardiovascular issues, and reproductive problems. Diagnosis involves clinical evaluation, blood tests for thyroid hormones (T3, T4, TSH), and imaging techniques such as ultrasound. Treatment depends on the underlying condition and may include hormone replacement therapy, antithyroid medications, radioactive iodine, or surgery. Timely diagnosis and proper management are critical to preventing complications, such as cardiovascular diseases and infertility. This abstract emphasizes the need for regular screening, especially in high-risk populations,

Keywords: *Thyroid disorders Hypothyroidism Hyperthyroidism Thyroiditis Goiter Hashimoto's thyroiditis*

Presented as Poster

Gender-Specific Insights On Metabolic Syndrome And Early Heart Failure Rehospitalization In Older Adults

Scan to View online

Presented by
G . Shreya Raj, Dr.B.Durga Pavan Kumar
Aditya Pharmacy College, Aditya University, Surampalem, Andhra Pradesh, India

Abstract

Metabolic syndrome (mets) and heart failure (hf) remain major global health challenges, impacting individuals of all age groups. These factors each play a role in higher rates of hf hospitalizations and early readmissions, emphasizing the need for clinical research and management in these key areas. It is crucial to understand the disparities between male and female patients with heart failure, especially when it comes to the risks of being readmitted to the hospital, in order to enhance the outcomes of these patients. The results emphasized the intricacy and variability of main risk indicators, such as gender-related differences, profiles of risk factors, and the efficacy of treatment approaches. Even though these risk factors are present before hf events, the exact impact they have on early rehospitalization (<60 days) is still not clear based on current data. Further research is needed to enhance risk estimation due to the common occurrence and serious outcomes of mets and repeat hf hospitalizations. A concerted effort is essential to close current disparities in hf research to uncover the impact of potential risk factors or their combinations on early (≤ 60-day) hf rehospitalization following an initial hf hospitalization, potentially with the help of a machine-learning strategy.

Keywords: *Heart Failure, Metabolic Syndrome, Rehospitalization, Gender – Specific.*

Presented as Poster

Drug Discovery And Regulatory Affairs, Drug Safety And Pharmacovigilance

Scan to View online

Presented by
K.Sanjana
VJ's College of Pharmacy, Rajahmundry, Andhra Pradesh, India

Abstract

The field of drug discovery and development is a multifaceted and dynamic process that encompasses various stages, each critical to the successful introduction of novel therapeutic agents to the market. The first section delves into the intricate landscape of drug discovery, highlighting the latest technological advancements, innovative approaches, and collaborative strategies that drive the identification and validation of potential drug candidates. The second segment of the abstract addresses' regulatory affairs, elucidating the pivotal role regulatory agencies play in shaping the drug development process. An examination of global regulatory frameworks and evolving guidelines provides insights into the challenges faced by pharmaceutical companies in navigating complex regulatory landscapes. The third thematic focus is on drug safety and pharmacovigilance, crucial components of post-market surveillance and risk management. Additionally, emerging trends in real-world evidence and the integration of big data analytics in pharmacovigilance practices are discussed. Overview of the interconnected processes that contribute to the successful development, approval, and monitoring of pharmaceutical products.

Keywords: *Dynamic, therapeutic, integrate, surveillance, pharmacovigilance*

Presented as Poster

Nanothernostics : A Promising Approach For Breast Cancer Diagnosis And Treatment Using Upconversion Nanoparticles

Scan to View online

Presented by
Nunna Iswarya, Nallamilli H.S.S.Chandana, Sadanala Satya Padmaja, Tellam Varshini
Aditya Pharmacy College, Aditya University, Surampalem, Andhra Pradesh, India

Abstract

Breast cancer is the most common cancer in women and a leading cause of cancer-related deaths worldwide. Early diagnosis and effective treatment are key to improving survival and quality of life for patients. Nanotheranostics, which combine diagnostic and therapeutic capabilities in a single platform, are emerging as promising tools for enhancing breast cancer care. This unique luminescence allows for deeper tissue penetration and reduced phototoxicity, making ucnps highly effective in *in vivo* applications. Ucnps can be engineered for multifunctional roles, including drug and gene delivery, photothermal therapy (ptt), and photodynamic therapy (pdt), all of which are critical in treating breast cancer. In drug delivery, ucnps can be functionalized with targeting ligands to enhance the precision of therapeutic agents, while in ptt and pdt, ucnps can facilitate localized tumor destruction through heat or reactive oxygen species generation upon nir light irradiation. Their ability to serve as both diagnostic imaging agents and therapeutic carriers offers a dual approach that is invaluable in cancer management. However, challenges such as toxicity, biocompatibility, and large-scale production remain, hindering their clinical translation. Continued research is necessary to optimize these nanomaterials and explore their full potential in breast cancer diagnosis and therapy.

Keywords: *Nanothernostics,Breast Cancer, Upconversion Nanoparticles (UCNPs),Rare Earth metals,Cancer diagnosis, Nanomedicine.*

Presented as Poster

Utilizing Cheminformatics In Addition To Other Methods For Efficient Natural Product Research

Scan to View online

Presented by
Y.Pallavi, Y.Sirisha
Aditya Pharmacy College, Aditya University, Surampalem, Andhra Pradesh, India

Abstract

For the development of new drugs, natural ingredients have provided a wealth of inspiration. However, it might take a lot of time and resources to do natural product research using conventional methods. An effective method for accelerating and streamlining natural product research is cheminformatics, or the application of computer and information technology to chemistry. With regard to the several facets of natural product research, this poster provides an extensive synopsis of cheminformatics software. Establishing the chemical structures of natural products by computer techniques is known as "structure elucidation.predicting molecular characteristics, including toxicity, lipophilicity, and solubility.creating models to relate molecular structures to biological activities is known as quantitative structure-activity relationship [qsar] modelling.analyzing and mining data: drawing insightful conclusions from big collections of information about natural products.. Compared to experimental techniques, cheminformatics tools can be more affordable. Potential drug candidates can be found by virtually screening natural product libraries using cheminformatics technologies. The quality and quantity if the data utilized to train cheminformatics tools determines their accuracy.

Keywords: *Cheminformatics, Natural Products, Virtual Screening, Data Mining, Structure Elucidation, Qsar, Affordable, Decreases Manual Labor.*

Presented as Poster

Ethanolic Leaf Extract Of Nymphea Stellata As An Antibacterial And Antiinflammatory Agent

Scan to View online

Presented by
S.Amala,Neelima,Mukesh
Aditya College of Pharmacy, Aditya University, Surampalem, Andhra Pradesh, India

Abstract

Medicinal plants are part and parcel of human society to combat diseases. They usually contain many biologically active ingredients and are used primarily for treating mild or chronic ailments. According to world health organization (who), about 80% of the world population relies chiefly on the plant based traditional medicine especially for their primary healthcare needs. Herbal medicines are in great demand because of their wide biological and medicinal activities, higher safety margins and lesser costs 3, 4. The present aim of the study is to prove of anti-microbial activity and anti-inflammatory activity of nymphaea stellata.to the methanol extract preliminary phytochemical screening was performed by using standard chemical tests. The methanol extracts of plant for its infectious and/or inflammatory nature were screened for *in-vitro* antibacterial and anti-inflammatory activities. The albino rats were used for acute toxicity studies as per oecd guidelines. The extracted compounds mebm, bme, bmc, bmh, bmq has been evaluated for their antimicrobial activity and anti-inflammatory activity. Antibacterial activity was tested using the agar diffusion method while anti-inflammatory activity was tested using the carrageen induced paw edema method. The zone of inhibition and anti-inflammatory was measured as per standard protocol which indicated the test showed significance results with standard drug.

Keywords: *Nymphaea Stellata Albino Rats, Oecd, Agar Diffusion, Antibacterial, Zone Of Inhibition*

Presented as Poster

Artificial Intelligence in Drug Discovery

Scan to View online

Presented by
N. Rohini Amrutha, S. Monali
VJ's College of Pharmacy, Rajahmundry,
Andhra Pradesh, India

Abstract

Drug discovery is a crucial area of research for pharmaceutical companies and scientists. However, the challenges during drug design and discovery are very high cost and long output time. Further, clinical trials in humans, microarray data, proteomics and genomics produce a big complex data. Artificial intelligence(AI) play a crucial role in drug discovery and development. In other words, artificial neural networks(ANN) and deep learning(DL) algorithms have simplified the drug discovery and development. The AI in drug discovery involves the process of drug design, polypharmacology, chemical synthesis, drug repurposing and drug screening. The present article provides a review on various AI tools and procedure involved in drug discovery such as predicting 3D structure of target protein, drug- protein interactions, determining drug activity, de novo drug design etc.

Keywords: *Artificial network, 3D structure, Target protein*

Presented as Poster

A Modern Manufacturing System Facilitates Pharmaceutical Operations

Scan to View online

Presented by
Y Sirisha, Y. Pallavi, V. Ambica Taruni
Aditya Pharmacy College, Aditya University, Surampalem, Andhra Pradesh, India

Abstract

The "lean manufacturing" ideology in pharmaceutical operations is primarily concerned with reducing or eliminating waste and increasing production with enhanced safety and efficacy. By implementing the four important lean principles like value stream mapping, just in time production, 5s, kaisen, and maintenance and total production. Initially value stream mapping enhances the production process by identifying and removing waste; just-in-time production focuses on promoting a lower-cost supply chain in increased demand situations; and 5s and kaisen are tools that organizes the workspace safe and clean to workspace while also encourages step-by-step continuous improvement. Moreover productive maintenance deals with overall equipment effectiveness, lowering the cost of equipment by preventing its breakdown. Higher output with fewer resources can be achieved through lean manufacturing's ability to increase productivity and may enhance customer satisfaction by meeting customer expectations and delivering items on schedule. Despite the many advantages of lean manufacturing, it's important to recognize some of its possible disadvantages, including initial investment, supply chain dependence, resistance to new change, lack of flexibility, and greater workload.

Keywords: *Eliminating Waste, 5S, Kaisen, Supply Chain, Value Stream Mapping,*

Presented as Poster

Personalized Cancer Vaccines

Scan to View online

Presented by
Ch.Angel , V.Kavya Sri , K.Sandhya Sri
VJ's College of Pharmacy, Rajahmundry,
Andhra Pradesh, India

Abstract

Tremendous innovation is underway among a rapidly expanding repertoire of promising personalized immune-based treatments. Therapeutic cancer vaccines (TCVs) are attractive systemic immunotherapies that activate and expand antigen-specific CD8+ and CD4+ T cells to enhance anti-tumor immunity. Our review highlights key issues impacting TCVs in clinical practice and reports on progress in development. We review the mechanism of action, immune-monitoring, dosing strategies, combinations, obstacles, and regulation of cancer vaccines. Most trials of personalized TCVs are ongoing and represent diverse platforms with predominantly early investigations of mRNA, DNA, or peptide-based targeting strategies against neoantigens in solid tumors, with many in combination immunotherapies. Multiple delivery systems, routes of administration, and dosing strategies are used. Intravenous or intramuscular administration is common, including delivery by lipid nanoparticles. The emerging trials illustrate the complexity of developing this class of innovative immunotherapies. Methodical testing of the multiple potential factors influencing immune responses, as well as refined quantitative methodologies to facilitate optimal dosing strategies, could help resolve uncertainty of therapeutic approaches.

Keywords: *Adjuvant; Cancer Immunotherapy; Clinical Pharmacology; Clinical Trials; Drug Development;*

Presented as Poster

Organ Regenerative Therapy An Overview

Scan to View online

Presented by
Karthik. M, Chaitnanya. L, D. Dileep, R. Amarnayak
VJ's College of Pharmacy, Rajahmundry, Andhra Pradesh, India

Abstract

New technologies consisting of stem cells and tissue-engineering have potential for augmenting organ function or repairing damaged organ. If explored to their full potential organ bio-engineering and regeneration technologies hold the promise to address two most urgent needs in organ transplantation, namely, the identification of a new, potentially inexhaustible source of organs and immunosuppression free transplantation of tissues and organs. A worldwide shortage of organs for clinical implantation establishes the need to bring forward and test new technologies that will help in solving the problem. The concepts of regenerative medicine hold the potential for augmenting organ function or repairing damaged organ or allowing regeneration of deteriorated organs and tissue. Researchers are exploring possible regenerative medicine applications in organ transplantation so that coming together of the two fields can benefit each other. Other organs (lung, pancreas, and intestine) are also routinely transplanted, although in less numbers. Groundbreaking achievements in regenerative medicine have generated interest in transplant researchers and they are exploring possible regenerative medicine applications in organ transplantation so that coming together of the two fields can benefit one another.

Keywords: *3D organ printing, Tissue Engineering, Clinical Transplantation, Bio-Engineering.*

Presented as Poster

Artificial Womb Technology

Scan to View online

Presented by
Moripi Yogitha, Devireddy Bindu Hasini
Srinivasa Rao College of Pharmacy,
Visakhapatnam, Andhra Pradesh, India

Abstract

Artificial womb technology, also known as ectogenesis, stands at the forefront of reproductive innovation, reshaping our understanding of conception, pregnancy, and childbirth. It is also known as artificial uterus technology as it grows a foetus outside the body and also helps premature babies develop and survive. This technology can potentially be performed as a switch from a natural uterus to an artificial uterus ,thereby moving the threshold of foetal vialability to a much earlier stage of pregnancy. The foundation of artificial womb technology lies in bioengineering where a controlled environment mimics the conditions of a natural womb. The fluid used in this technology mimics amniotic fluid. This technology is a potential solution for surrogacy. This innovation allows for the gestation of embryos outside the human body, offering new possibilities for couples struggling with infertility, premature births, and high-risk pregnancies. This technology has the potential to reduce maternal mortality rates, eliminate the risk of prenatal exposure to harmful substances, and promote gender equality by sharing the responsibilities of childbirth more equitably. Artificial womb technology represents a paradigm shift in Gynaecology.

Keywords: *Ectogenesis, surrogacy, infertility,extrauterine system , artificial uterus,bioartificial uterus.*

Presented as Poster

Stem Cells:Pioneering The Future Of Drug Development

Scan to View online

Presented by
M.Akshaykumar,G.Chandraleka,Md.Salma,Y.Keert hi
School of Pharmaceutical Sciences & Technologies, JNTU, Kakinada, Andhra Pradesh, India

Abstract

Stem cells are unspecialised cells of human body.They are able to differentiate into any cell of an organism and have ability to self renewal. Stem cells exist both in embryo and adult. Stem cells have great potential to become one of the most important aspects of medicine. In addition to fact that they play a large role in developing restorative medicine, their study reveals much information about the complex events that happen during human development. Stem cell as a target for pharmacological testing.stem cell based drug delivery system evolved against problems like insufficient targetting and undesirable treatment efficiency Stem cells can be in new drug tests. Each experiment on living tissue can be performed safely on specific differentiated cells from pluripotent cells. Due to this technique,it can become possible to generate healthy heart muscle and later transplant them to patients with heart diseases. With each experiment, the capabilities of stem cells are growing, although there are still many obstacles to overcome. Tissue banks are becoming more nowadays as they gather cells that are the source of the regenera tive medicine in a struggle against present and future diseases. With stem cell therapy and all its regenerative benefits, we are better able to prolong human life than any time in history.

Keywords: *Stem cells ,Pharmacological testing , restorative medicine,stem cells based drug delivary ,regenerative benefits ,therapy for disease, tissue banks*

Presented as Poster

Quality-Driven Optimization Of Hydrogel Systems Incorporating Clitoria Ternatea Extract

Scan to View online

Presented by
Divya Narla, Velagala Urmila, Sana Sai, S Jhansi Lakshmi
Aditya College of Pharmacy, Aditya University, Surampalem, Andhra Pradesh, India

Abstract

The flowers of clitoria ternatea were known for their broad range of health benefits owing to their rich profile of phytochemicals. They exhibit antioxidant, anti inflammatory, anti cancer, cognitive enhancement and many other properties. In the present work the benefits of antioxidant and anti inflammatory properties were harnessed into a topical hydrogel to provide anti aging effect in conjuction with moisture retention. Quality by design approach was used to formulate hydrogels and the optimization was done by 32 factorial design using design expert software. Combination of natural and synthetic gelling agents such as carbopol 934 & guar gum were used for preparing hydrogels. The optimized formulation was further evaluated for various parameters such as ph, spreadability, microbial growth, stability tests, skin irritation and hydration tests. The optimized formulation exhibited 65.5 % scavenging activity against dpph reflecting its antioxidant property and the skin hydration enhanced from 36% to 41.4% without causing any irritation.

Keywords: *Quality By Design, Design Expert Software, Topical Hydrogel, Antiageing*

Presented as Poster

Aquasomes:Vesicular Drug Delivery

Scan to View online

Presented by
Vyshnavi P, Jyothsna
Aditya Pharmacy College, Aditya University, Surampalem, Andhra Pradesh, India

Abstract

Aquasomes are a new type of drug delivery system specilised to improve how medications work in our body. They have special structure consists of core made of sugars or other substances surrounded by protective outer layer. This model allows aquasomes to catch both water-loving (hydrophilic) and water-repelling (hydrophobic) drugs, making them versatile for various types of medications.the main benefits of aquasomes is that they can help less dissolve soluble drugs, which is common problem in medicine. By enhancing solubility, aquasomes ensure that more of the drug is absorbed by our body, leading to better treatment results. The outer layer can also be modified to target specific cells, such as cancer cells, which helps deliver the medication exactly where it's needed and reduces side effects.aquasomes can be designed to release their drug in response to changes in the body, like ph levels or temperature. It means that the drug can be released at the right time and place, increasing its effectiveness.aquasomes offer a promising strategy to drug delivery by improving solubility, targeting, and controlled release. They have the potential to make treatments more effective and safer for patients. As research continues,aquasomes play a significant role in advancing specilised medicine and improving healthcare result across different diseases

Keywords: *Aquasomes, hydrophobic, hydrophilic solubility,drug delivery*

Presented as Poster

3D Printing In Pharmaceutics : Revolutionizing Drug Formulation And Delivery

Scan to View online

Presented by
Vyshnavi Penaganti
Aditya Pharmacy College, Aditya University, Surampalem, Andhra Pradesh, India

Abstract

This article explains how 3d printing, also known as additive manufacturing, is changing the way we create medications. With respect to traditional methods there can be slow and hard, 3d printing allows for quick and simple designing of drugs for individual patients. Doctors can combine more medications into one drug, making it easier for patients to take their drug as prescribed. It looks into dissimilar 3d printing techniques, like stereolithography, combined deposition modeling, and selective laser sintering. Each technique has its own strengths, like creating precise shapes and improving how the medicine is released in the body. Some 3d-printed tablets dissolve quickly, others release medication over a longer time. This technology can produce medications in just one step, which reduces waste and enhances treatment effectiveness. In 3d printing for healthcare grows, holds great promise for innovating how we develop and deliver medications. It leads to better health outcomes, as patients receive drugs designed exactly for their needs. Overall, 3d printing is covering the way for a future where medicines are more unique, making healthcare morelacking and improving patients' lives. This innovative approach streamlines production, reduces costs, and enhances patient compliance, paving the way for transformative healthcare advancements.

Keywords: *3D Printing,Additive Manufacturing,Drug Formulation, Medication Delivery,Healthcare Innovation*

Presented as Poster

Mouth Dissolving Tablets

Scan to View online

Presented by
K Naveena, N Kamakshi,N Bannu
Raghu College of Pharmacy,
Bheemunipatnam, Andhra Pradesh, India

Abstract

Mouth-dissolving tablets (MDTs), also known as orally disintegrating tablets (ODTs), are a type of fast-dissolving medication designed to dissolve or disintegrate quickly in the mouth without the need for water. Developed to improve patient compliance and ease of administration, especially for populations with swallowing difficulties (like pediatric and geriatric patients), MDTs utilize specialized formulations that allow for rapid breakdown upon contact with saliva. This rapid dissolution ensures a faster onset of action compared to traditional tablets, making them suitable for medications requiring prompt therapeutic effects, such as analgesics or antihistamines. MDTs are prepared through various methods, including freeze-drying, spray drying, and direct compression.Emerging innovations continue to refine the formulation and production of MDTs, making them a growing sector within pharmaceutical development aimed at enhancing patient experience and compliance across various therapeutic areas.

Keywords: *Disintegrants,dissolvents,mouth dissolving tablets, antihistamines,analgesic, medication*

Presented as Poster

Accelerating Drug Discovery Through Artificial Intelligence And Collaboration

Scan to View online

Presented by
M.G.V.S. Krishnam, Sree Lakshmi Adhikari, Md Farhana, Dr. K.Purna Naga Sree
Raghu College of Pharmacy, Bheemunipatnam, Andhra Pradesh, India

Abstract

The integration of AI into drug discovery and development has revolutionized the pharmaceutical industry, enhancing precision and efficiency across the drug development pipeline. AI's application spans crucial stages such as target identification lead compound discovery, and clinical trials, significantly reduced the time and cost associated with traditional method. Notable examples include DSP-1181 and INSO18_055 for obsessive-compulsive disorder, developed by Exscientia and Sumitomo Dainippon Pharma, and Barucitinib, repurposed for COVID-19 treatment by BenevolentAI. Key AI tools like convolutional neural networks. (CNNs), recurrent neural networks (RNNs)(CNNs), recurrent neural networks (RNNs), and natural language processing (NLP) are explored for their specific applications in pharmaceutical research. Despite significant advancements, challenges such as data quality, algorithm transperancy, and the need for interdisciplinary collaboration remain. Addressing these issues is crucial for regulatory approval and broader acceptance in the scientific community, AI integrated drugs discovery promises to accelerate innovation, reduce costs, and improve therapeutic success rates, provided current challenges are effectively managed and interdisciplinary collaboration is embraced.

Keywords: *Artificial Intelligence, Drugs Discovery, Pharmaceutical Industry, AI integration, Machine learning, Deep learning, Challenges and Solutions.*

Presented as Poster

Formulation And Evaluation Of Verapamil Hydrochloride Fast Dissolving Tablets By Using Natural Super Disintegrant Ocimum Gratissimum Seed Mucilage Powder

Scan to View online

Presented by
G. Sai Sandhya
Aditya College of Pharmacy, Aditya University, Surampalem, Andhra Pradesh, India

Abstract

Verapamil hydrochloride is a calcium channel blocker used to treat hypertension and angina fast dissolving tablets offer improved patient compliance and natural super disintegrants like ocimum gratisimum seed mucilage powder can replace synthetic ones and the methods which are used are the extraction of mucilage powder from ocimum gratisimum seeds and the formulation of fast disintegrants using different concentration of mucilage powder and then they are combined with the verapamil and evaluation tests were carried out such as disintegration time, dissolution time, hardness , content uniformity, friability, invitro release studies and the results are carried out well at different concentrations when these tests are carried out such as disintegration time, hardness, dissolution rate ,. And content uniformity and finally ocimum gratisimum has proved as natural super disintegrant for verapamil hydrochloride enhancing patient compliance and potentially reducing side effects.

Keywords: *Fast Dissolving Tablets, Verapamil Hydrochloride, Ocimum Gratissium Mucilage, Natural Super Disintegrant*

Presented as Poster

Pharmacoeconomics And Pharmacoepidemiology In The Pharmaceutical Field

Scan to View online

Presented by
Chekuri.Niharika, M. Saraswathi,
G.Anusha Durga
VJ's College of Pharmacy, Rajahmundry,
Andhra Pradesh, India

Abstract

Together, pharmacoeconomics and pharmacoepidemiology are evaluating the overall worth of pharmaceuticals in the healthcare system. By integrating economic evaluations with epidemiological data, these fields support the development of evidence-based guidelines and policies, ultimately aiming to improve patient outcomes and optimize healthcare expenditures. There are combined with advancing quality, safety, and efficiency of drug therapies. These analysis the economic aspects of pharmaceutical sciences. It impacts on public health and Education, it also underscore the critical role in these two fields in optimizing healthcare delivery, enhancing patient outcomes and ensuring the efficient use of cost management and resources. These use the effects of drugs in large populations. It combines principles of epidermiology and clinical pharmacology to understand the model, motives and effects of medication use. Pharmacoeconomics focuses on assessing the economic impact of drug therapies, including their cost-effectiveness, cost-utility, and costbenefit. On other hand, pharmacoepidemiology evaluates the templates, reasons and effects of drug use in large populations.

Keywords: *Epidemiology data, Healthcare syastem, cost-utility, cost-effective treatment, monitoring drug safety, effect of drug on patients, economic impacts of drug therapies*

Presented as Poster

Bridging The Gaps In Neuro Perception

Scan to View online

Presented by
N.Svd Krishna Sri,D.B Satya Sai Sri Lakshmi,K.Tejaswini,P.Gangothri
School of Pharmaceutical Sciences & Technologies, JNTU, Kakinada, Andhra Pradesh, India

Abstract

The concept of bridging the gap in neuro perception focuses on combining therapeutic, surgical, and artificial interventions to restore or enhance human sensory abilities. Sensory perception encompassing sight, hearing, touch, and other senses is often compromised by injury, disease, or congenital conditions. medical approaches like surgery and therapy play a vital role in repairing damaged sensory pathways. Advances in neurostimulation, and rehabilitation strategies have enhanced the ability to restore sensory functions. These devices, powered by advancements in artificial intelligence (AI), neural networks, and robotics, allow for more naturalistic sensory input by closely mimicking biological systems. AI algorithms can help improve auditory clarity, visual recognition, and tactile sensitivity in these devices. Such approaches aim not only to restore lost functions but also to create seamless, human-like experiences through the combination of biological and technological means. This multidisciplinary strategy has the potential to dramatically enhance the quality of life for individuals with sensory disabilities, by offering solutions that span both medical intervention and cutting-edge technology, reducing the gap between human and artificial sensory perception.

Keywords: *Sensory perception, advanced surgery techniques, artificial devices, natural therapy*

Presented as Poster

Neuralink In Paralysis

Scan to View online

Presented by
B.Ruth Blessy, R. Harshitha
VJ's College of Pharmacy, Rajahmundry, Andhra Pradesh, India

Abstract

Neuralink is an american company that is developing implantable brain computer interfaces (BCI) .The companies goal is to implant electrode polymer chips into human brain to connect them directly to machines. This would help people suffering from diseases like paralysis and parkinsons disease by allowing communication between the brain and external devices. Neuralink plans to develop a small chip that can read thousands of brain signals per second and connect the brain wirelessly to computers to provide benefits like deep brain stimulation and potentially enhance human abilities over time. The chip aims to allow paralyzed people to walk again by communicating with a chip below an injured spinal cord .However there are also risks like safety and technical hurdles to overcome before this technology can be used widely in humans. This review article explores about Advantages, disadvantages, benefits to patients and potential of neuralink in treating aliments.

Keywords: *Neuralink, Polymer chips, Paralysis, Parkinson's disease,Brain computer*

Presented as Poster

Encouraging People With Diabetes And Chronic Kidney Disease To Optimize Their Finerenone: A Pharmacist'S Opportunity

Scan to View online

Presented by
Dr. D.V.S Somayajulu, Lalitha Maheswari Dandipati, Hima Bindu Gudimettla, Pushpa Satya Mahalakshmi Sanivarapu
Aditya Pharmacy College, Aditya University, Surampalem, Andhra Pradesh, India

Abstract

CKD, especially in the type 2 diabetic patient, is a disease that needs to be managed and dealt with carefully to avoid further complications. to this end, drugs such as finerenone, showing an effect that reduces nonsteroidal mineralocorticoid receptor antagonism-associated risks, force their prescribers, pharmacists, to be part of multidisciplinary care teams. A literature review on the role of pharmacists in the management of ckd, and finerenone optimization, is done. it explores the analyses that involve pharmacist-led interventions, identification of patients for use of finerenone, the adjustments in the therapy, and finally monitoring drug efficacy and safety. Pharmacists play a role in identifying the eligible patients through screening tests, ensuring proper dosing, monitoring renal function and potassium levels, and managing drug interactions. education and counseling improve patient adherence for better outcomes. however, caution should be exerted in the use of finerenone therapy because of risks, such as hyperkalemia, particularly among patients being treated with concurrent medications influencing potassium balance. In the multidisciplinary management of the ckd patients on finerenone, pharmacists play an important role, and ultimately, contribute to improved patient outcomes by ensuring that medications are adhered to in a safe and effective manner.

Keywords: *Finerenone, Nonsteroidal Mineralocorticoid Receptor, Hyperkalemia, Albuminuria, Optimization, Antagonism-Associated Risks.*

Presented as Poster

Human Endoceuticals : A New Era In Drug Research

Scan to View online

Presented by

Agnitha Christeena Geddam; Devi Sravanthi Yamala; Sai Prasanna Divya Tanniru

Sir C. R. Reddy College of Pharmaceutical Sciences, Eluru, Duggirala, Andhra Pradesh, India

Abstract

Human endoceuticals are bioactive compounds designed to enhance, regulate, or modulate the body's natural processes. This presentation explores various forms, including hormone replacement therapy, monoclonal antibodies, cytokine therapies, gene therapies, stem cell therapies, etc., And also it explains about how endoceuticals differ from traditional pharmaceuticals and how they aim to optimize physiological functions at a cellular or molecular level. The advantages of endoceuticals include reduced side effects, biocompatibility,personalized medicine, targeted treatment, long-term efficacy, and diverse applications. However, challenges such as high costs, complex manufacturing processes, potential immune reaction etc., Each approach gives the body's innate biological systems to promote healing and restore balance, addressing a wide array of conditions from hormonal deficiencies to cancer and regenerative challenges, illustrating about wound healing, cancer, HIV and other neurological disorders. Human endoceuticals also promise for advancing therapeutic strategies in modern medicine, utilizing the body's mechanisms to develop effective treatments that could revolutionize patient care. Continued research is essential for realizing their full potential and ensuring safe, accessible therapies for diverse health conditions.

Keywords: *Bioactive compounds, Regenerative Medicine, Personalized Medicine, Targeted therapies, Biocompatibility, Optimized cellular processes*

Presented as Poster

Nanotechnology : Shaping The Future Of Drug Delivery System

Scan to View online

Presented by
Dhanusri Bhupathi
Aditya Pharmacy College, Aditya University, Surampalem, Andhra Pradesh, India

Abstract

Nanotechnology is making medicine delivery better. It helps doctors send the right dose of drug to the target place in our bodies. This decreases harm to healthy cells and makes treatments more accurate. Small particles known as nanoparticles are used to carry medicine to target areas. This helps treating the diseases like cancer, alzheimer's, and infections more effectively. Researchers are working to make this technology safer and more available. Their aim is to create personalized treatments that work better for each patient. With nanotechnology, medicine will become more accurate ,effective, and easier to take and safe. Nanotechnology in medicine has even more benefits. Smaller doses are needed, making treatment more effective. This could lead to treatments for before untreatable diseases and improved vaccine capability. Nanotechnology is transforming healthcare, making medicine more precise, unique, and life-changing. Small particles called nanosensors detect biomarkers for diseases like cancer, allowing for timely treatment. This technology also leads to quicker recovery times, decreased hospital stays, increased patient comfort, more effective wound healing, and improved dental care. Overall, nanotechnology transforms healthcare, offering new hope for patients and increasing quality of life.

Keywords: *Nanotechnology, Medicine Delivery, Targeted Therapy, Alzheimer'S Disease , Nanoparticles.*

Presented as Poster

Stem Cell Therapy In The Treatment Of Cancer

Scan to View online

Presented by
Prasanna Mohan
VIgnan Institute of Pharmaceutical Technology, Visakhapatnam, Andhra Pradesh, India

Abstract

The study on 'stem cell therapy on the treatment of cancer' is currently under pre clinical trials is the new emerging scope for the cure of cancer. Despite the advancements in research and technology, the cancer death rate has only declined by 1.5% between 2019-20 in US. Various treatment of radiotherapy, chemotherapy,surgical removal of solid tumor and immunotherapy for cancer end up with various ADRs like therapeutic resistance and cancer recurrence. The Stem Cell(SC) possess biological actions like self renewal ,differentiation , migration and modulation of neighbouring cells, hence used as regenerative medicine, drug targeting and immune generation against cancer cells . Stem cells including Pluripotent Stem Cells(PSCs), Haematopoietic Stem Cells(HSCs), human Mesenchymal Stem Cells(hMSCs) each with varying properties can be used for targeted action on the tumor microenvironment, cancer cell migration,tumor angiogenesis, proliferation and differentiation of affected cells. SCs have high proliferative action however their limited lifespan in *In vivo* culture conditions acts as an obstacle for their clinical applications (e.g: hMSCs have short lifespan). Highly targeted action of the Stem Cells(SCs) estimated to provide more efficient results compared to current methods of cancer treatment. The various mechanisms they adopt during Intravenous infusion helps study its detailed pharmacology.

Keywords: *Cancer, Stem cell,In vivo,Targeted action, Tumor Micro environment*

Presented as Poster

Biosensors For Drug Safety And Delivery

Scan to View online

Presented by
Karthik , Vijaya , Durga , Aruna
Viswanadha Institute of Pharmaceutical Sciences, Sontyam, Visakhapatnam, Andhra Pradesh, India

Abstract

Biosensor-integrated drug delivery systems are innovative devices in the health area, enables the continuous monitoring and drug administration. The use of smart polymer, bioMEMS, and electrochemical sensors have been extensively studied for these systems, especially for chronic diseases such as diabetes mellitus(DM), cancer and cardiovascular diseases(CVD) as well as advances in regenerative medicine. Basically, the technology involves sensors designed for the continuous analysis of biological molecules followed by drug release in response to specific signals. The advantages include high sensitivity and fast drug release. In this work, the main advances of biosensor-integrated drug delivery systems as new biomedical materials to improve the patients quality of life with chronic diseases are discussed.

Keywords: *Biosensors , Drug delivery systems , Smart polymers , Bio-medical applicaions , Chronic treatments.*

Presented as Poster

Alphafold - The Future Of Structure-Based Drug Design

Scan to View online

Presented by
Pardha Saradhi Yedida , Shaik Sayed Salman
School of Pharmaceutical Sciences & Technologies, JNTU, Kakinada, Andhra Pradesh, India

Abstract

The ability to predict protein structures has been a bottleneck in the process of drug discovery as it limits the scope of finding drugable targets. This is the case of AlphaFold which is a breakthrough in the prediction of protein structures, but still poses some questions on its application in drug design processes, especially in the prediction of binding sites and interactions with ligands. In this report the utility of AlphaFold is examined in practical terms by way of its predictions being incorporated in linear drug development processes that are already in existence, in this case, molecular docking and ligands' binding site determination. The structures of the AlphaFold models were compared to their experimental counterparts yielding an average RMSD of less than 1.5 Å. Moreover, it boosted the owned percentage success rates in virtual screening by 25% and excellent results were also recorded when predicting the allosteric sites, extending the scope of drug discovery. Owing to the provision of protein structures, AlphaFold enhances drug design processes by reducing the need for experimental methods like X-ray crystallography. It assists in the initial stages of drug design, especially when experimental data is absent.

Keywords: *Drug development, RMSD(Root mean square deviation), Molecular docking, AlphaFold, Drug discovery, X RAY Crystallography.*

Presented as Poster

Kuru Disease

Scan to View online

Presented by
G. Amulya, M. Pushpa Latha
VJ's College of Pharmacy, Rajahmundry, Andhra Pradesh, India

Abstract

Kuru is a neurodegenerative disorder caused by a misfolded prion protein that replicates and accumulates in the brain leading to brain damage and eventual death. The name kuru means "to shiver" or "trembling in fear". Kuru disease also known as "Laughing Sickness" is a rare and infections prion disease that affected the indigenous people of Papua New Guinea, particularly the fore tribe. The epidemic finally declined sharply after half a century, from 200 deaths per year in 1957 to no deaths from at least from at least 2010 onwards, but sources disagree on whether the last known kuru victim died in 2005 or 2009.Majorly 60% cases are seen females and 2% cases are seen adult males and 38% cases are seen children of both sexes. This review article explores about pathophysiology, etiology, potential treatment for disease.

Keywords: *Cannibalism, Laughing Sickness, Prion Proteins, Seizures*

Presented as Poster

Innovative Learning: Digital Tools In Pharmaceutical Education

Scan to View online

Presented by
V.Bhavana, Md.Farheena, V.Sirisha
VV Institute of Pharmaceutical Sciences,
Gudlavalleru, Andhra Pradesh, India

Abstract

Pharmacists have faced the biggest challenges ever experienced in the history of the profession: the use of digital technologies in pharmacy practice and education, as well as the outbreak of coronavirus disease 2019. The use of digital technologies in pharmaceutical care has dramatically increased globally and will add to patient care. The use of digital technologies in pharmacy education has been dramatically increased and incorporated into the teaching- learning process. Hence, in this new era of pharmacy practice and education, curricula should focus on developing specific skills in the cognitive, conscious, and efective use of digital tools. This implies the training of "disruptive" n eslsecers, equipped to adopt teaching-learning methods conditioned by the digital environment and education processes appropriate to foster effective disruptive technology use. The commentary concludes that the pharmacy profession cannot afford to wait for slow integration of digital technologies in pharmacy practice and education.

Keywords: *Augmented reality, computer-assisted instruction,digital technology , patient simulation,virtual reality*

Presented as Poster

Evaluating Mental Well-Being And Resilience In Kakinada'S Elderly: Insights From A Community-Based Cross-Sectional Study

Scan to View online

Presented by
Manikanta Reddy Vatrapu, Abburi Sri Satya Shinney, Pavan Kumar Yanamadala
Aditya Pharmacy College, Aditya University, Surampalem, Andhra Pradesh, India

Abstract

Health and mental well-being problems, the need to increase healthcare assistance, and the quality of life for the elderly are just a few of the areas that have been significantly impacted by kakinada's shift to a pensioner's paradise in recent years. Investigating the physical and emotional well-being of the elderly in kakinada society is therefore crucial. A community-based cross-sectional study was carried out to evaluate the mental and physical well-being of senior citizens living in kakinada. From june-august of 2024, 174 samples in all were gathered from the kakinada district. The basic geriatric screening (bgs) and the mental well-being quality of life questionnaires (mhqol) were used to gather data. Additionally, the questionnaire on demographic variables was used. The data was analyzed using descriptive statistics. 67.4% of the 174 samples in total were female. We took into account the participant's age group of 60-85 years. The subjects had a 64.0% prevalence of chronic illnesses. A nutritional status evaluation showed that, according to bmi, 52.0% of the individuals were underweight. According to disability data, 72.4% of participants reported issues with their oral well-being, 65.8% had eye impairments, and 12.2% had hearing impairments. In general, 22.7% of the elderly had poor mental well-being, and 9.4% had difficulties in their daily life activities. The findings indicated that mental well-being, disability, and non-communicable diseases were the main well-being issues affecting the elderly.

Keywords: *Mental well-being, Elderly, Resilience, chronic illnesses.*

Presented as Poster

AI-Driven Innovations In Pharmacy: Shaping The Future Of Healthcare

Scan to View online

Presented by
Yeturi Sravanthi,Nadisetti Sandhya
Aditya Pharmacy College, Aditya University, Surampalem, Andhra Pradesh, India

Abstract

Artificial intelligence (AI) is a set of technologies that allow computers to perform tasks that mimic human intelligence, such as seeing, understanding language and analysing data. The integration of artificial intelligence in pharmaceutical industry enhancing efficiency and accuracy in various stages of the process. Ai accelerates the identification of potential drug candidates, optimizes clinical trial designs, and improves patient stratification. The integration of ai - driven predictive analytics helps in assessing drug safety and efficacy, thereby reducing time and costs associated with bringing new therapies to market. Ai has been employed in medical fields including radiology, pathology, cardiology, dermatology. In radiological imaging, ai excels at detecting fractures, tumors with high precision. Pathologists benefit from ai in identifying cancerous cells, while cardiologists use it to predict heart disease risk. Dhermatologists use ai to recognize skin conditions from images. Further more, ai enhances the design of clinical trials by identifying patient populations, predicting outcomes and monitoring safety signals. Ai holds the potential to significantly reduce the time and cost associated with bringing new therapeutics to market, innovative treatments and personalised medicine.

Keywords: *Drug Development, Drug Discovery, Patient Outcomes, Preclinical Testing, Treatment Response Prediction.*

Presented as Poster

Xenotransplantation

Scan to View online

Presented by
Maddirala Gracy Suguna
Srinivasa Rao College of Pharmacy,
Visakhapatnam, Andhra Pradesh, India

Abstract

Xenotransplantation using pigs as the transplant source has the potential to resolve the severe shortage of human organ donors. Although the development of relatively non-toxic immunosuppressive or tolerance-inducing regimens will be required to justify clinical trials using pig organs, recent advances in our understanding of the biology of xenograft rejection and zoonotic infections, and the generation of α1,3-galactosyltransferase-deficient pigs have moved this approach closer to clinical application. Organ allotransplantation has now reached an impassable ceiling inherent to the limited supply of human donor organs. In the United States, there are currently over 100,000 individuals on the national transplant waiting list awaiting a kidney, heart, and/or liver transplant. This is in contrast with only a fraction of them receiving a living or deceased donor allograft. Given the morbidity, mortality, costs, or absence of supportive treatments, xenotransplant has the potential to address the critical shortage in organ grafts. Last decade research efforts focused on creation of donor organs from pigs with various genes edited out using CRISPR technologies and utilizing non-human primates for trial. Three groups in the United States have recently moved forward with trials in human subjects and obtained initial successful results with pig-to-human heart and kidney xenotransplantation.

Keywords: *xenotransplantation, kidney, heart, liver, clinical trial, xenograft*

Presented as Poster

Transforming Nephrology In India: The Role Of Women And Win-India Initiatives

Scan to View online

Presented by
Hepzibah Rani Gidla, Dr. D. V. S. Somayajulu, Dr. Pavan Kumar Yanamadala
Aditya Pharmacy College, Aditya University, Surampalem, Andhra Pradesh, India

Abstract

The establishment of women in nephrology-india (win-india) marks a significant advancement in the effort to combat gender inequality within the field of nephrology and to foster a more inclusive healthcare system in india. Founded in 2021, win-india serves as a professional network that empowers female nephrologists through various means, including mentorship, educational opportunities, and advocacy initiatives. This review explores the diverse roles that win-india plays in promoting gender equity in nephrology, highlighting how the unique insights and experiences of women can enhance patient care and contribute to a more inclusive healthcare landscape. Through initiatives such as online seminars, symposia, and the #iwinchat discussions, win-india facilitates knowledge exchange and professional development, benefiting both seasoned nephrologists and those at the beginning of their careers. The organization also tackles challenges within the workplace by advocating for fair compensation, mental health resources, and family-oriented policies, thereby highlighting its dedication to achieving a healthy work-life balance. Through initiatives such as mentorship programs, community outreach, and continuous research, win-india empowers women in the field of nephrology, enabling them to make significant contributions to innovative kidney care while fostering a legacy of excellence and inclusivity.

Keywords: *Women in Nephrology, Gender Diversity, WIN-India, Healthcare Leadership, Patient Advocacy, Kidney Health, Medical Mentorship, Nephrology*

Presented as Poster

The Impact Of Educational Structures On Nursing Competency In India And Developed Nations

Scan to View online

Presented by

Hepzibah Rani Gidla, Mrs. Mahalakshmi Dasi, Dr. Pavan Kumar Yanamadala
Aditya Pharmacy College, Aditya University, Surampalem, Andhra Pradesh, India

Abstract

Nursing education is crucial in healthcare, significantly impacting patient outcomes and care quality. In india, aspiring nurses can begin their education after secondary school, pursuing either a diploma or a bachelor of science in nursing (bsn) after twelve years of formal schooling. Conversely, in more developed nations like the united states and canada, entry into nursing programs necessitates higher academic prerequisites, including foundational courses in biology and chemistry, to ensure that students possess a solid grounding in the basic sciences. The duration of nursing programs also varies; indian diploma courses typically last three years, while bsn programs extend to four years, aligning with the duration of similar programs in the united states and canada. However, the curricular focus diverges significantly: Indian nursing education tends to emphasize fundamental care skills, whereas curricula in developed countries prioritize evidence-based practice, critical thinking, and leadership competencies. This disparity is further reflected in the clinical training requirements and faculty qualifications; developed nations often mandate more extensive clinical placements and require faculty to hold advanced degrees, such as master's or doctoral qualifications, to facilitate evidence-based teaching and research. Additionally, the differences in licensing requirements contribute to the professional landscape, as developed countries enforce stringent examinations and speciality certifications, thereby upholding high standards across various nursing specialties.

Keywords: *Nursing Education, Curriculum Comparison, India, Developed Countries, Patient Care Outcomes, Faculty Qualifications*

Presented as Poster

Revitalizing Traditional Medicines: The Resurgence Of Herbal Drugs In Modern Days

Scan to View online

Presented by
Md.Sameena, N.Sravani ,Pr.Sravya Sri, T.Mahitha
Raghu College of Pharmacy, Bheemunipatnam, Andhra Pradesh, India

Abstract

Herbal medicine, one of the oldest forms of healthcare, remains a pivotal element in global health systems, especially in modern integrative and alternative medicine. In modern healthcare, herbal remedies are being validated through clinical studies and standardized for therapeutic use, leading to greater acceptance among medical practitioners and patients. In recent years, many herbal compounds have been identified as effective against chronic diseases, inflammatory conditions, and mental health disorders. The demand for natural, sustainable treatments is driving the popularity of plant-based formulations, particularly in areas such as oncology, immunology, and metabolic disorders. However, challenges such as variability in herb quality, adulteration, regulatory gaps, and potential drug-herb interactions present barriers to integration into mainstream medicine. Proof of safety and effectiveness needed for issuing manufacturing licenses for different categories of ASU (Ayurvedic, Siddha, and Unani) drugs is mentioned in Rule 158B of the Drugs & Cosmetics Rules, 1945. Herbal drug analysis using modern analytical techniques such as High-performance liquid chromatography (HPLC), High-performance thin layer chromatography(HPTLC), High-performance thin layer chromatography - Mass spectroscopy (HPTLC-MS), Liquid Chromatography - Mass Spectroscopy (LC-MS) has thus become indispensable in ensuring the quality, efficacy, and safety of herbal medicines, supporting their growing role in integrative healthcare.

Keywords: *Herbal medicine, Ayurvedic pharmacopoeia, Standardization, Quality control, Analytical techniques*

Presented as Poster

Internal Validation Of Tecan Freedom Evo 75 Robot

Scan to View online

Presented by
Chinnimilli Harshitha , Kurella Venkata Mani Kavya , Somireddy Jayasri
Lydia College of Pharmacy, Ethakota, Ravulapalem, Andhra Pradesh, India

Abstract

The tecan freedom evo 75 is a device that is used for pipetting small volumes. The Fredom evo 75 has been developed to handle repetitive handling tasks and can be utilized either independently or in conjunction with an analytical system. Before. using your method on the robot, you can test it with the Freedom Evo SIM TM 3D stimulation tool. Creating a new technique in this manner prevents you from tying up your instrument. Semi- or fully automated Elisa can be highly cost-effective when using the 8 plus 1 access pipetting arm of the Tecan Freedom Evo 75. On the other side of detailed research and to capture your assay running in a 3D simulation, you can use the Freedom Evo SIM. While Compared with instruments, the technology eliminates the tedious steps of adding reagents by more than 80%. However, the technology has exceptional repeatability from a single point. Even For a 1 ul volume, the technique can be reproduced with outstanding accuracy and is advantageous for automated in-situ hybridization.

Keywords: *Automated Process, Insitu Hybridisation , Pipetting Of Small Volumes,Cost Effective , 3d Simulation , Elisa , Pre Validation*

Presented as Poster

The Role Of AI In Drug Discovery

Scan to View online

Presented by
G.Rishiitha Raj , S.Vyshnavi
Koringa College of Pharmacy, Korangi, Tallarevu (M), Andhra Pradesh, India

Abstract

Artificial intelligence (AI) has the potential to revolutionize the drug discovery process, offering improved efficiency, accuracy, and speed. However, the successful application of AI is dependent on the availability of high-quality data, the addressing of ethical concerns, and the recognition of the limitations of AI-based approaches. In this article, the benefits, challenges, and drawbacks of AI in this field are reviewed, and possible strategies and approaches for overcoming the present obstacles are proposed. The use of data augmentation, explainable AI, and the integration of AI with traditional experimental methods, as well as the potential advantages of AI in pharmaceutical research, are also discussed. Overall, this review highlights the potential of AI in drug discovery and provides insights into the challenges and opportunities for realizing its potential in this field. Note from the human authors: This article was created to test the ability of ChatGPT, a chatbot based on the GPT-3.5 language model, in terms of assisting human authors in writing review articles. The text generated by the AI following our instructions (see Supporting Information) was used as a starting point, and its ability to automatically generate content was evaluated. After conducting a thorough review, the human authors practically rewrote the manuscript, striving to maintain a balance between the original proposal and the scientific criteria. The advantages and limitations of using AI for this purpose are discussed in the last section.

Keywords: *Artificial intelligence, drug discovery, AI-assisted content generation, AI-limitations*

Presented as Poster

Cardiovascular Kidney Metabolic Syndrome

Scan to View online

Presented by
T Sai Sri Mounika,B.Aprna
VJ's College of Pharmacy, Rajahmundry, Andhra Pradesh, India

Abstract

The correlation between obesity, type 2 diabetes mellitus (DM), cardiovascular disease (CVD), and chronic kidney disease (CKD) is an escalating and widely acknowledged epidemic in industrialized nations. Recently, this complex web of interrelated health conditions has been collectively defined as the Cardiovascular-Kidney-Metabolic (CKM) syndrome by the American Heart Association (AHA). The molecular mechanisms underlying CKM disease contain a spectrum of interconnected factors, including hyperglycemia, insulin resistance, heightened activity of the renin-angiotensin-aldosterone system (RAAS), the generation of advanced glycation end-products, oxidative stress, lipotoxicity, endoplasmic reticulum stress, abnormalities in calcium handling, malfunctioning of mitochondria and impaired energy production, as well as persistent chronic inflammation. Addressing their prevention, management, and treatment is of paramount importance to promote better patient health outcomes. The objective of this review is to provide a comprehensive and critical examination of the current state-of-the-art regarding the recently defined CKM syndrome. This includes an exploration of epidemiological evidence establishing connections between cardio-renal-metabolic diseases, an examination of the underlying pathophysiological mechanisms, and a comprehensive overview of existing treatment modalities.

Keywords:*Diabetes mellitus (DM) , Cardiovascular disease(CVD) , Chronic kidney disease (CKD) , Obesity , American Heart Association (AHA)*

Presented as Poster

Natural 3D-Printed Stem Cells For Wound Healing And Tissue Regeneration

Scan to View online

Presented by
Mandapati Sravanthi, Kothapalli Sujitha Sri, Komma Pushpa Poojitha, Dalli Santoshi
Srinivasa Rao College of Pharmacy, Visakhapatnam, Andhra Pradesh, India

Abstract

Wound healing is a natural process that occurs when the body replaces tissue with new tissue. It involves many cell types, mediators, cytokines and vascular system. The wound healing process has 3 phases. 1. Inflammation 2. Proliferation 3.Remodeling. This latest techniques involved in wound healing are revolutionizing the way we treat injuries and promote recovery. The latest technique used is 3D-printing stem cells technique. The 3D-printed tissue engineered skin substitutes have shown remarkable results in accelerating wound healing. These 3D printed stem cells are involved in wound healing, reducing inflammation and improving tissue regeneration. These are involved in decellularized adipose tissue with the anti-inflammatory property by using Celecoxib (COX-2). These also determine the formation of stable 3D porous network structure that supports cell growth. This wound-healing process is carried among the skin burns and their treatment over the 3D printing stem cells technique on the surface of skin. This content indicates the anti-microbial, anti-bacterial and anti-inflammatory activities among the COX-2 drugs, which majorly helps in reducing the inflammation. This poster helps to gain knowledge on the 3D-printing technique for wound healing,along with the process of formation of different layers of medication on the wounds in detail.

Keywords: *3D- printing stem cells, Reduction of inflammation, Tissue Regeneration, Anti-inflammatory property, Celecoxib (COX-2) material, Risk of infection.*

Presented as Poster

Utilizing Cheminformatics In Addition To Other Methods For Efficient Natural Product Research.

Scan to View online

Presented by
Y.Pallavi,Y.Sirisha
Aditya Pharmacy College, Aditya University, Surampalem, Andhra Pradesh, India

Abstract

For the development of new drugs, natural ingredients have provided a wealth of inspiration. However, it might take a lot of time and resources to do natural product research using conventional methods. An effective method for accelerating and streamlining natural product research is cheminformatics, or the application of computer and information technology to chemistry. With regard to the several facets of natural product research, this poster provides an extensive synopsis of cheminformatics software. We will talk about the potential use of cheminformatics tools in to find the possible medication candidates from big databases of natural products are known as virtual screening. Establishing the chemical structures of natural products by computer techniques is known as "structure elucidation. "predicting molecular characteristics, including toxicity, lipophilicity, and solubility. Creating models to relate molecular structures to biological activities is known as quantitative structure-activity relationship [QSAR] modeling. Compared to experimental techniques, cheminformatics tools can be more affordable. Potential drug candidates can be found by virtually screening natural product libraries using cheminformatics technologies. The quality and volume of data used to train cheminformatics tools determines their accuracy. For particular research needs, it is crucial to carefully evaluate the limitations and select the appropriate tools.

Keywords: *Cheminformatics, Natural Products, Virtual Screening, Data Mining, Structure Elucidation, Qsar, Affordable.*

Presented as Poster

Unlocking Adipose Potential

Scan to View online

Presented by
B.Shamili Sree
VJ's College of Pharmacy, Rajahmundry,
Andhra Pradesh, India

Abstract

Diabetes management necessitates innovative solutions to address insulin deficiency. Utilizing advanced cellular reprogramming techniques, biocompatible scaffolding, and stem cell biology, we investigate the potential of differentiating adipocytes into functional pancreatic beta-like cells. The study employs a combination of genetic engineering, growth factor manipulation, and micro environmental conditioning to enhance the efficiency of this conversion process. Preliminary results indicate a promising yield of insulin-secreting cells that exhibit glucose-responsive behaviour, suggesting their viability for therapeutic applications. *In-vitro* and *in vivo* experiments reveal a significant increase in insulin production, responsiveness to glucose, and improved metabolic regulation. This work not only contributes to the field of regenerative medicine but also offers a novel approach to tackling insulin deficiency in diabetic patients, potentially leading to ground breaking advancements in diabetes care. Key findings reveal the underlying mechanisms of adipocyte plasticity and the role of specific signalling pathways in promoting beta-cell differentiation, laying the groundwork for future clinical applications. This review paper explores about innovative methodologies for converting adipose (fat) tissues into insulin-producing cells, addressing a critical need in diabetes treatment and management.

Keywords: *Diabetes, Insulin deficiency, Adipose tissue, Cellular reprogramming, Biocompatible Scaffolding, Stem cell biology, Regenerative medicine.*

Presented as Poster

The Power Of AI In Herbal Drug Development And In Silico Screening For Natural Product Leads

Scan to View online

Presented by
Bhavyasri Nandipati, N.Srisusmitha,
P.Chandini, P.Ahammadunnisa, G.Sowjanya
Aditya Pharmacy College, Aditya University,
Surampalem, Andhra Pradesh, India

Abstract

Natural product discovery is accelerated by ai/ml, which also optimizes lead compounds and predicts bioactivity. Molecular docking, qsar, and deep learning are some of the methods. Computational techniques predict bioactivity and find lead compounds by analyzing the structure-activity connections of natural products. By forecasting binding affinity and efficacy, in silico screening and docking find possible natural product leads. Docking software (autodock, glide) and molecular modeling tools (pymol, visual molecular dynamics) are used in in silico screening. Complex links and possible leads are revealed by the integration and analysis of herbal medicine data using big data and bioinformatics. Techniques include network analysis and data mining. Ai-powered molecular docking predicts binding affinity and efficacy, optimizing plant-based medication development. Integrating omics data (genomics, proteomics, and metabolomics) offers a thorough comprehension of pharmacognostic substances. Potential natural product leads are found using virtual screening techniques that forecast bioactivity and efficacy. Deep learning algorithms predict the toxicity and efficacy of medicinal plants by identifying their bioactive components. Natural drug discovery is being transformed with the integration of computational technologies in pharmacoinformatics. The authenticity and uniformity of herbal drugs are guaranteed by next-generation sequencing and computer-aided analysis.

Keywords: *Natural Products, AI, Molecular Docking, Molecular Modelling Tools, Deep Learning Algorithm, Next-Gen Sequencing.*

Presented as Poster

Chemi Informatics

Scan to View online

Presented by
K John Wesley
Viswanadha Institute of Pharmaceutical Sciences, Sontyam, Visakhapatnam, Andhra Pradesh, India

Abstract

The intricate architecture of the biomolecules that cause diseases like AIDS, cancer, autism, AIDS, and AIDS, among others, make it difficult for medical researchers to find medications to treat them. Due to changes in a number of elements, such as dietary habits, environmental conditions, and migration in human lifestyles, it is now essential to design and create new, effective anti-drugs for diseases that do not cause adverse consequences. Cheminformatics focuses on finding pharmaceuticals using contemporary drug discovery methods, which address intricate problems in conventional drug discovery systems. Medical chemists can better comprehend the intricate structures of chemical substances with the use of cheminformatics technologies. The primary goal of the newly developing interdisciplinary discipline of cheminformatics is to find novel chemical entities.[NCE] that eventually leads to the creation of a novel molecule [chemical data]. It is also crucial for gathering, preserving, and evaluating chemical data. In order to help chemists and medical researchers solve complex diseases, this study focuses on cheminformatics and its applications in drug discovery as well as contemporary drug discovery approaches.

Keywords: Chemi informatics, AIDS, Drug discovery.

Presented as Poster

Natural Antibiotics Against Antimicrobial Resistance

Scan to View online

Presented by
Kadiyala Yamini Swapna, A. Jyothi Prasanna, J. Akshaya Durga
VJ's College of Pharmacy, Rajahmundry, Andhra Pradesh, India

Abstract

Drug-resistant bacteria pose a serious threat to human health worldwide. Current antibiotics are losing efficacy and new antimicrobial agents are urgently needed. Living organisms are an invaluable source of antimicrobial compounds. The antimicrobial activity of the most representative natural products of animal, bacterial, fungal and plant origin are reviewed in this paper. Their activity against drug-resistant bacteria, their mechanisms of action, the possible development of resistance against them, their role in current medicine and their future perspectives are discussed. Natural compounds of heterogeneous origins have been shown to possess antimicrobial capabilities, including against antibiotic-resistant bacteria. The most commonly found mechanisms of antimicrobial action are related to protein biosynthesis and alteration of cell walls and membranes.

Keywords: *Natural antimicrobial, antimicrobial resistance, phytochemicals, polyphenols*

Presented as Poster

Innovative Learning; Digital Tools In Pharmaceutical Education

Scan to View online

Presented by
V.Sirisha , Md.Farheena Sulthana , V.Bhavana
VV Institute of Pharmaceutical Sciences, Gudlavalleru, Andhra Pradesh, India

Abstract

Pharmacists have faced the biggest challenges ever experienced in the history of the profession: the use of digital technologies in pharmacy practice and education, as well as the outbreak of coronavirus disease 2019. The use of digital technologies in pharmaceutical care has dramatically increased globally and will add to patient care. The use of digital technologies in pharmacy education has been dramatically increased and incorporated into the teaching- learning process. Hence, in this new era of pharmacy practice and education, curricula should focus on developing specific skills in the cognitive, conscious, and efective use of digital tools. This implies the training of "disruptive" neslsecers, equipped to adopt teaching-learning methods conditioned by the digital environment and education processes appropriate to foster
effective disruptive technology use. The commentary concludes that the pharmacy profession cannot afford to wait for slow integration of digital technologies in pharmacy practice and education.

Keywords: *Augmented reality, Computer-assisted instruction, Digital technology, Patient simulation, Virtual reality*

Presented as Poster

Developing And Applying Photoplethysmography In Pharmacy

Scan to View online

Presented by
N. Rohith Sai, D. Lokesh Naga Likhith, S.Mahesh, T Harika
School of Pharmaceutical Sciences & Technologies, JNTU, Kakinada, Andhra Pradesh, India

Abstract

Photoplethysmography is an optical, non-invasive technique to sense the variations in blood volume in microvascular tissue. That's commonly known as photoplethysmography or PPG. PPG detects changes in light absorption and reflection caused by pulsatile blood flow, enabling the extraction of crucial information about physiological factors such as heart rate and, importantly, blood oxygen saturation (SpO2) and other cardiovascular health markers. The technique usually uses a light source, like an LED, and a photodetector, which records the light that is reflected or transmitted ppg has become widely used because of its affordability, ease of use, and simplicity, which make it appropriate for continuous monitoring in a variety of contexts, including clinical settings and wearable technology that transitions from the clinical to the mobile world. Other benefits include pulse oximetry.

Keywords: *Non-invasive, Capable of continuous monitoring, Portable equipment, low-cost, photoplethysmography*

Presented as Poster

Therapeutic Potential Of Clitoria Ternatea (Ct) Flower In Managing Poly Cystic Ovary Syndrome (PCOS): Effects On Obesity Reduction

Scan to View online

Presented by
Md.Rawoof
VJ's College of Pharmacy, Rajahmundry,
Andhra Pradesh, India

Abstract

The aim of this study was to know about the overview of the Clitoria Ternatea (CT) flower in treatment of poly cystic ovarian syndrome (PCOS) by decreasing the weight of an individual by its anti obese property and some other therapeutic uses, by decreasing the mental stress towards it. The crude drug / phytopharmaceutical Clitoria Ternatea (CT) flower was selected for this study. It is prepared by the extraction technique by using various types of extraction solvents (ethanol, methanol, ethyl acetate, and hexane). In India; recommends for the treatment of the snake and scorpion bites of the clitoria ternatea extract stem. The main phytoconstituents found in CT flower extract are anthocyannins and tannins. So these Phytoconstituents has the potential to act as the anti diabetic, anti obesity, anti- oxidant, antiglucose, anticholesterol activities. It is also a treatment of the diuretic, laxative and atherosclerosis. The main potential in this study is about the Anti-obese property. This study provided an insightful overview of Clitoria Ternatea (CT) flower and its potential therapeutic applications, particularly in the treatment of poly cystic ovarian syndrome (PCOS). The focus was on its anti-obese properties and other therapeutic uses aimed at reducing weight and alleviating mental stress associated with PCOS.

Keywords: *Anthocyannins, Clitoria ternatea, PCOS*

Presented as Poster

Pill Cam - Capsule Endoscopy

Scan to View online

Presented by
M Sangeetha,M Durga Srija, R Sowjanya, V Bhavana
Sri Vasavi Institute of Pharmaceutical Sciences, Pedatadepalli, Andhra Pradesh, India

Abstract

-Advances in fields like nanotechnology. Gene therapy has the potential to completely transform how we find and create medications as well as how we identify and treat illnesses. One new invention that is attracting a lot of curiosity is the "camera in a pill." Only the proximal (esophagus, stomach, and duodenum) and distal (colon) parts of the gastrointestinal tract were readily accessible with current technology until recently. It was virtually impossible to reach the twenty feet or so of small intestine that separated these two sections. Colonoscopy or endoscopy. The gastrointestinal (GI) tract can be seen with a non-invasive diagnostic procedure called a capsule endoscopy, or cam pill. You ingest a tiny camera that resembles a pill. A recording device worn on your body receives the thousands of photographs it takes as it passes through your digestive system. This approach is especially helpful for inspecting regions, such as the small intestine, that may be difficult for standard endoscopy to access. Investigations into problems including Crohn's disease, unexplained GI bleeding, and other small intestinal disorders are frequently conducted using it.

Keywords: *Nanotechnology,Crohn's disease, endoscopy,small intestine*

Presented as Poster

Epigenetic Alterations In Cancer

Scan to View online

Presented by
V. Geethika, K.T.V.M.Amrutha
VJ's College of Pharmacy, Rajahmundry, Andhra Pradesh, India

Abstract

Epigenetic mechanisms are essential for normal development and maintenance of tissue-specific gene expression patterns in mammals. Disruption of epigenetic processes can lead to altered gene function and malignant cellular transformation. Global changes in the epigenetic landscape are a hallmark of cancer. The initiation and progression of cancer, traditionally seen as a genetic disease, is now realized to involve epigenetic abnormalities along with genetic alterations. Recent advancements in the rapidly evolving field of cancer epigenetics have shown extensive reprogramming of every component of the epigenetic machinery in cancer including DNA methylation, histone modifications, nucleosome positioning and non-coding RNAs, specifically microRNA expression. The reversible nature of epigenetic aberrations has led to the emergence of the promising field of epigenetic therapy, which is already making progress with the recent FDA approval of three epigenetic drugs for cancer treatment. In this review, we discuss the current understanding of alterations in the epigenetic landscape that occur in cancer compared with normal cells, the roles of these changes in cancer initiation and progression, including the cancer stem cell model, and the potential use of this knowledge inindesigning more effective treatment strategies.

Keywords: *Epigenetics, cancer,hypoxia, DNA methylation ,histone modification, mRNAs, chromatin*

Presented as Poster

Computational Modelling Of Drug Response With Application To Neuroscience

Scan to View online

Presented by
K. Mounika Lakshmi, J. Yamini, Sania
VJ's College of Pharmacy, Rajahmundry, Andhra Pradesh, India

Abstract

The development of novel high-throughput technologies has opened up the opportunity to deeply characterize patient tissues at various molecular levels and has given rise to a paradigm shift in medicine towards personalized therapies. Computational analysis plays a pivotal role in integrating the various genome data and understanding the cellular response to a drug. Based on that data, molecular models can be constructed that incorporate the known downstream effects of drug-targeted receptor molecules and that predict optimal therapy decisions. In this article, we describe the different steps in the conceptual framework of computational modeling. We review resources that hold information on molecular pathways that build the basis for constructing the model interaction maps, highlight network analysis concepts that have been helpful in identifying predictive disease patterns, and introduce the basic concepts of kinetic modeling. Finally, we illustrate this framework with selected studies related to the modeling of important target pathways affected by drugs

Keywords: *bioinformatics; drug response; dynamic modeling; molecular interaction; network analysis; neurogenomics; systems biology.*

Presented as Poster

Theranostics:Combining Theraphy And Diagnostics For Personalized Medicine

Scan to View online

Presented by
Sirapurapu Manjula
Aditya Pharmacy College, Aditya University, Surampalem, Andhra Pradesh, India

Abstract

Theranostics is a word that is used to combines treatment and diagnosis to improve ones healthcare. This process increases precise identification and targeted treatment of diseases, leading to better patient outcomes. Theranostics uses advanced and accurate technologies like tiny particles, genetic markers, and artificial intelligence to tailor treatment to individual needs. It has shown promise in some treatments like cancer, neurological disorders, heart conditions, and infections. Theranostics gives several profits, which includes accurate diagnosis with more effective treatment along with fewer side effects, real-time monitoring, and improved patient outcomes. While there are challenges, ongoing research aims to overcome these problems and make theranostics more accessible. Theranostics also gives some additional profits including personalized medicine tailored to genetic profiles, decreased healthcare costs through targeted interventions, increased patient engagement and empowerment, and streamlined clinical trials and drug development. Its potential applications extend to some rare diseases and pediatrics. Future research plans on advancing nanotechnology and biomaterials, integrating artificial intelligence and machine learning, and developing point-of-care theranostic devices and instruments.furthermore, theranostics is expected to strech to new disease areas, addressing regulatory and reimbursement challenges

Keywords: *Theranostics,Targeted Therapy, Diagnostics, Nanotechnology, Artificial Intelligence,Healthcare,Revolution,Point-Of-Care Devices*

Presented as Poster

Sleep Role In The Dark Struggle; Unravelling The Link Between Nightmares And Addictions.

Scan to View online

Presented by
B. Subbu Rao, M. Haritha, P. Manga Raju
Viswanadha Institute of Pharmaceutical Sciences, Sontyam, Visakhapatnam, Andhra Pradesh, India

Abstract

Steroids and various drugs are known to cause sleep disturbances, including insomnia, by influencing the central nervous system and hormonal rhythms. Corticosteroids, commonly prescribed for inflammatory conditions, interfere with the body's natural production of cortisol, leading to heightened alertness and difficulty falling asleep. This disruption can be especially pronounced when steroids are taken at higher doses or in the evening. Additionally, certain classes of medications, such as stimulants (including caffeine, amphetamines, and some weight-loss drugs) and specific antidepressants, can have stimulating effects on the brain, making it challenging to initiate and maintain sleep. These drugs increase levels of neurotransmitters like dopamine and norepinephrine, elevating alertness and arousal. The consequences of drug-induced insomnia can be severe, impacting mental and physical health by contributing to fatigue, decreased cognitive function, and an increased risk of chronic health issues like hypertension and depression. Individuals on long-term steroid or stimulant regimens may face ongoing sleep disturbances, emphasizing the need for careful management. Healthcare providers should monitor patients for signs of insomnia and explore potential adjustments in medication timing, dosage, or even alternative treatments when appropriate. Behavioral approaches, such as cognitive-behavioral therapy for insomnia (CBT-I), can also provide valuable support, helping to mitigate sleep disturbances and improve quality of life.

Keywords: *steroids, drug abuse, insomnia, cognitive function, hormones*

Presented as Poster

Tuberous Sclerosis In Adult Patients: Clinical Insights And Management For A 39-Year-Old Female

Scan to View online

Presented by
Manikanta Reddy Vatrapu, Abburi Sri Satya Shinney, Pavan Kumar Yanamadala
Aditya Pharmacy College, Aditya University, Surampalem, Andhra Pradesh, India

Abstract

Tuberous sclerosis complex (tsc) is a genetic disorder caused because of mutations in the tsc1 or tsc2 genes, forming hamartomas in many organs, including the skin, brain, eyes, kidneys, heart, and lungs. It is believed that these genes stop cells from developing too fast or uncontrollably. The sort of symptoms in tsc is distinctive: may include as angiofibromas and hypomelanotic macules, neurological (seizures, developmental delays), and renal complications (angiomyolipomas). While it is mostly diagnosed in childhood, adults can also develop the ailment and other complications. This case report details the diagnosis, treatment options, and clinical symptoms of a 39-year-old patient with tsc. Cutaneous lesions were the patient's initial manifestations, in conjunction with recurrent seizures and renal angiomyolipomas diagnosed through imaging studies. A multidisciplinary team approach was therefore employed, related to physicians from the departments of dermatology, neurology, and nephrology. Management consisted of anticonvulsant therapy to reduce the seizures as well as monitoring of the renal characteristic so that it will gauge the need for possible surgical intervention based on the scale and range of renal tumours. This case report brings out the significance of diagnosing tsc in adults and management tailor-made at the know-how that the disorder evolves with time. Considering the multiple manifestations of the disease, regular screenings and specialised treatment plans are essential for quality care.

Keywords: *Tuberous Sclerosis Complex, Hamartomas, Angiofibromas, Hypomelanotic Macules, Seizures, Angiomyolipomas.*

Presented as Poster

Targeting DNA Repair To Combat Cancer Chemo Resistence

Scan to View online

Presented by
Pulagam Bharath,Tarigoppala Saivenkat,Vaddi Aditya,Vipparala Manoj
Sri Vasavi Institute of Pharmaceutical Sciences, Pedatadepalli, Andhra Pradesh, India

Abstract

Cancer ranks as the second leading cause of death following heart disease. However, considering the increase in its incidence, cancer is expected to take over first place in causes of death within the next 10–15 years. Despite major advances in medicine, we still have not achieved the desired results in the treatment of cancer. Cancer chemoresistance, the ability of tumor cells to evade the cytotoxic effects of chemotherapy, is a major obstacle in successful cancer treatment. One of the key mechanisms underlying chemoresistance is the enhanced capacity of cancer cells to repair DNA damage caused by chemotherapeutic agents. DNA repair pathways, such as homologous recombination (HR), non-homologous end joining (NHEJ), and base excision repair (BER), play a critical role in maintaining genomic stability. However, in cancer cells, these pathways are often upregulated or mutated, enabling rapid repair of chemotherapy-induced DNA lesions, leading to survival and resistance. Combining DNA repair inhibitors with traditional chemotherapy or radiotherapy may enhance the therapeutic response by exacerbating DNA damage and preventing repair. This abstract outlines the importance of targeting DNA repair mechanisms as a therapeutic approach to overcome cancer chemoresistance and highlights the potential of combination therapies to improve clinical outcomes.

Keywords: *Cancer chemoresistence,targeting DNA,combination therapies,clinical outcomes,application*

Presented as Poster

Spinal Muscular Atropy

Scan to View online

Presented by
Alugu Alpha, M.Kavya Kusuma
VJ's College of Pharmacy, Rajahmundry,
Andhra Pradesh, India

Abstract

SMA is one of the genetic disease. It is characterized by the muscle weakness and atrophy. SMA is autosomal recessive neuro muscular disease characterized by degeneration of motor neuron in spinal cord. It primarily affects infants and children. Recent advanced treatment particularly gene therapy and SMA modulators are used to treat the SMA patient. About 1 get affected in 6000 to 10,000 births. Individuals suffering with SMA have the common complications like scoliosis, hip dislocation and joint contractures. One in fifty people carry a copy of the altered gene that can lead to SMA in child. Nerve cells that controls muscle are mostly located in the spinal cord. Symptoms that displayed at the birth of children has the lowest level of functions. The goal of SMA therapy is to increase the expression levels of the survival motor neuron protein at the right time in the correct cells. To increase the production of survival motor neuron several drugs are used. In this presentation we provide a comprehensive review that integrates clinical manifestations, therapeutic development, diagnostic strategy, molecular pathogenesis. This review will take a historical perspective to highlight important milestones in the travelling to developing effective therapies of SMA

Keywords: *SNA, Chromosome 5,gene therapy,hypotonia, ZOLGENSIMA, WERDNIG Hoffman disease*

Presented as Poster

Nipah Virus: A Zoonotic Threat To Global Health

Scan to View online

Presented by
Komala Aiswarya Kokku, J Bhargava Narendra
Aditya Pharmacy College, Aditya University, Surampalem, Andhra Pradesh, India

Abstract

A type of viral infection brought on by the nipah virus is called a nipah virus infection. It is an rna virus belonging to the "henipa virus" genus. Some "fruit bats" are typically the carriers of the virus. Niv is a bat-borne pathogen (zoonotic virus) that can infect humans directly or through contaminated food, causing fatal encephalitis. A range of illnesses, from asymptomatic infections to fever, cough, headache, dyspnea, serious respiratory infections and deadly encephalitis, are brought on by the virus. Approximately 50 to 75 percent of infected individuals die, and they may go into coma within a day or two. First identified in malaysia in 1998, the niv was discovered in siliguri, india, in 2001. It was then linked to a second outbreak in the nadia district of west bengal in 2007, and the current outbreak in kerala claimed over 17 lives and afflicted several others. Brain inflammation and seizures after healing are examples of complications. In most cases, physical contact with an infected source is necessary for spread. The diagnosis is made based on the patient's symptoms and verified by laboratory tests such as rt-pcr, phylogenetic analysis, serologic analysis, and niv sequencing. As of 2024, there is no licensed treatment or vaccination; therefore, management is limited to supportive care. Avoiding bats and sick pigs, as well as avoid drinking raw date palm sap, are preventive strategies.

Keywords: *Henipa Virus, Zoonotic Virus, Date Palm Sap, Encephalitis.*

Presented as Poster

The Pharmacological Promise Of Venom-Derived Peptides In Treating Neurological Disorders

Scan to View online

Presented by
Haritha.M, Y.V. Davan, K.Namratha
Viswanadha Institute of Pharmaceutical Sciences, Sontyam, Visakhapatnam, Andhra Pradesh, India

Abstract

This study explores the therapeutic potential of venom-derived peptides in treating neurological disorders such as Alzheimer's and Parkinson's diseases. Animal venoms, from sources like snakes, spiders, and marine species, contain bioactive peptides capable of selectively targeting key neural receptors and ion channels. These peptides exhibit neuroprotective, anti-inflammatory, and analgesic properties, making them ideal candidates for managing neurodegeneration. The main aim of this research is to evaluate the pharmacological mechanisms and efficacy of these venom peptides in mitigating neuronal damage and preserving cognitive function. With their specificity and reduced risk of side effects, venom-derived peptides offer an innovative approach to neurotherapeutics. In conclusion, venom-based pharmacology holds promise for the development of novel, effective treatments for complex neurological disorders, bridging nature's biochemistry with clinical applications.

Keywords: *1. Venom-derived peptides 2. Neuroprotection 3. Neurological disorders 4. Ion channels 5. Neuroinflammation 6. Neurodegenerative diseases*

Presented as Poster

Role Of AI In Uncover Therapeutic Uses Of Existing Drugs

Scan to View online

Presented by
S. Sirisha , K .Vyshnavi , N .Bavana , R. Spurthi Rekha.
Viswanadha Institute of Pharmaceutical Sciences, Sontyam, Visakhapatnam, Andhra Pradesh, India

Abstract

Artificial intelligence (AI) and machine learning, a subset of AI, are increasingly used in medicine. AI excels at performing well-defined tasks, such as image recognition; for example, classifying skin biopsy lesions, determining diabetic retinopathy severity, and detecting brain tumors. This article provides an overview of the use of AI in medicine and particularly in respiratory medicine, where it is used to evaluate lung cancer images, diagnose fibrotic lung disease, and more recently is being developed to aid the interpretation of pulmonary function tests and the diagnosis of a range of obstructive and restrictive lung diseases. The development and validation of AI algorithms requires large volumes of well-structured data, and the algorithms must work with variable levels of data quality. It is important that clinicians understand how AI can function in the context of heterogeneous conditions such as asthma and chronic obstructive pulmonary disease where diagnostic criteria overlap, how AI use fits into everyday clinical practice, and how issues of patient safety should be addressed. Overall, AI is expected to play a key role in aiding clinicians in the diagnosis and management of respiratory diseases in the future, and it will be exciting to see the benefits that arise for patients and doctors from its use in everyday clinical practice.

Keywords: *Asthma , Artificial intelligence , COPD Diagnosis , Machine learning ,Respiratory disease*

Presented as Poster

Ai In Breast Cancer Care: Enhancing Accuracy And Personalized Treatment

Scan to View online

Presented by
P.Manmadha Rao, B.Raja Rajeswari, R.Swathi
Aditya Pharmacy College, Aditya University, Surampalem, Andhra Pradesh, India

Abstract

Breast cancer is a significant cause of cancer-related mortality in women worldwide, and early, precise diagnosis is crucial for improving clinical outcomes. The rise of artificial intelligence (ai) has ushered in a new era in breast cancer care, notably in image analysis, leading to advancements in diagnosis and personalized treatment regimens. Ai transforms the diagnostic workflow by integrating machine learning algorithms for screening, diagnosis, staging, biomarker evaluation, prognostication, and therapeutic response prediction. Although traditional methods face challenges, including false positives, negatives, human errors, and time-consuming processes, ai-driven algorithms analyze complex data, recognize patterns, and provide accurate insights. Numerous studies show that ai performs equivalently or better than human readers. The ibrisk (intelligent-augmented breast cancer risk calculator) tool can predict whether abnormal tissue flagged by doctors is benign or cancerous. Ai also enables personalized treatment plans by analyzing genetic and molecular data, optimizing treatment effectiveness, and reducing adverse effects while aiding in surgical precision during tumor resection. The innovative integration of ai promises to revolutionize breast cancer screening and treatment strategies by overcoming human limitations and achieving remarkable precision. However, challenges remain in fully adopting ai clinically, underscoring the importance of focused research to realize ai's full potential in patient care.

Keywords: *Artificial Intelligence 1, Ibrisk Tool 2 ,Diagnostic Imaging 3, Pathology, Precision Medicine 4.*

Presented as Poster

Bilosomes Novel Drug Delivery System

Scan to View online

Presented by
D.Vijaya Lakshmi, G.Raga Surekha ,
Lakshmi Surekha
Aditya College of Pharmacy, Aditya University, Surampalem, Andhra Pradesh, India

Abstract

Bilosomes as a novel drug delivery system.bilosomes emerging as a novel vesicular drug delivery system,offering significant advantages in the delivery of bioactive molecules, especially via oral route.struturally, bilosomes are lipid based vesicles composed of bile salts and phospholipids,designed to improve the stability and encapsulated drugs or vaccines.by incorporation of bile salts imparts additional stability to the vesicles, allowing them to resist the harsh gastrointestinal environment, including the acidic ph of the stomach and enzymatic degradation. This stability enhences the delivery of the drugs or antigens to the small intestine, promoting better absorption and therapeutic efficacy. Bilosomes have shown great potential in improving oral vaccine formulations, particularly are that are typically degraded in the gastrointestinal tract. They are also being explored for the oral delivery of the peptides, proteins and other hydrophilic drugs that generally have poor bioavailability.

Keywords: *Bilosomes, Drug Delivery, Bioavailability, Bile Salts, Oral Vaccines.*

Presented as Poster

Artificial Intelligence In Pharmaceutical Technology And Drug Delivery Desighn

Scan to View online

Presented by
Yangala Swathi, Alluri.Venkatalakshmi
VJ's College of Pharmacy, Rajahmundry, Andhra Pradesh, India

Abstract

Artificial intelligence (AI) has emerged as a powerful tool that harnesses anthropomorphic knowledge and provides expedited solutions to complex challenges. Remarkable advancements in AI technology and machine learning present a transformative opportunity in the drug discovery, formulation, and testing of pharmaceutical dosage forms. By utilizing AI algorithms that analyze extensive biological data, including genomics and proteomics, researchers can identify disease-associated targets and predict their interactions with potential drug candidates. This enables a more efficient and targeted approach to drug discovery, thereby increasing the likelihood of successful drug approvals. Furthermore, AI can contribute to reducing development costs by optimizing research and development processes. Machine learning algorithms assist in experimental design and can predict the pharmacokinetics and toxicity of drug candidates. Personalized medicine approaches can be facilitated through AI algorithms that analyze real-world patient data, leading to more effective treatment outcomes and improved patient adherence. This review provides an overview of various AI-based approaches utilized in pharmaceutical technology, highlighting their benefits and drawbacks. Nevertheless, the continued investment in and exploration of AI in the pharmaceutical industry offer exciting prospects for enhancing drug development processes and patient care.

Keywords: *Artificial intelligence (AI), machine learning, drug discovery, formulation, dosage form testing, pharmacokinetics, pharmacodynamics, PBPK, QSAR*

Presented as Poster

Nanotheranostics: A Promising Approach For Breast Cancer Diagnosis And Treatment Using Upconversion Nanoparticles

Scan to View online

Presented by
Nunna Iswarya, Nallamilli Sri Chandana, Sadanala Satya Padmaja, Tellam Varshini
Aditya Pharmacy College, Aditya University, Surampalem, Andhra Pradesh, India

Abstract

Breast cancer is the most common cancer in women and a leading cause of cancer-related deaths worldwide. Early diagnosis and effective treatment are key to improving survival and quality of life for patients. Nanotheranostics, which combine diagnostic and therapeutic capabilities in a single platform, are emerging as promising tools for enhancing breast cancer care. Among these, rare earth metal-doped upconversion nanoparticles (UCNPS) have gained significant attention due to their ability to convert near-infrared (NIR) light into visible or ultraviolet (UV) light. This unique luminescence allows for deeper tissue penetration and reduced phototoxicity, making ucnps highly effective in *in vivo* applications. In drug delivery, ucnps can be functionalized with targeting ligands to enhance the precision of therapeutic agents, while in ptt and pdt, ucnps can facilitate localized tumor destruction through heat or reactive oxygen species generation upon nir light irradiation. Their ability to serve as both diagnostic imaging agents and therapeutic carriers offers a dual approach that is invaluable in cancer management. However, challenges such as toxicity, biocompatibility, and large-scale production remain, hindering their clinical translation. Continued research is necessary to optimize these nanomaterials and explore their full potential in breast cancer diagnosis and therapy.

Keywords: *Nanothernostics, Breast Cancer, Upconversion Nanoparticles (UCNPs), Rare earth metal, Cancer diagnosis, Nanomedicine.*

Presented as Poster

The Future Of Cervical Cancer:Role Of Pharmacists And Artificial Intelligence In Prevention And Management

Scan to View online

Presented by
Jyothsna Mamidi,Ganga Mahalakshmi Yenuganti, Sangeetha Palaka
Srinivasa Rao College of Pharmacy, Visakhapatnam, Andhra Pradesh, India

Abstract

Cervical cancer is the fourth leading cause of cancer related deaths among women worldwide. In 2022, 6.6 million new cases and 3.5 deaths were reported as per UNICEF data, indicating the seriousness of the disease. Cervical cancer originates in the epithelial filling of the cervix, the lower part of the uterus. Persistent infection with certain strains of human papillomavirus (HPV) leads to the development of cervical neoplasia. There are 130 types of mortal papillomavirus (HPV), belonging to the family of papillomaviridae, of which around 20 are associated with cancers of the anogenital tract and other mucosal areas. Screening programs and HPV vaccination can significantly reduce the incidence rate. Cervical cancer diagnosed at an early stage leads to 5-year survival rate of 91%. The Government of India conducts Programme called the cervical cancer National Breast & Cervical Cancer Early-Stage Detection Programme for awareness. A pharmacist can play a vital role in educating patients on HPV vaccination and screening, managing chemotherapy related adverse effects, optimising treatment outcomes and advocating for cervical cancer prevention and control policies. Artificial intelligence can help in developing predictive modeling for cancer risk assessment, personalised medicine using genomics and machine learning.

Keywords: *Cervical cancer, Pharmacist, Artificial intelligence, Human papilloma virus (HPV)*

Presented as Poster

Anesthesia In Heart Transplantation: Evolving Standards For Complex Care

Scan to View online

Presented by
Hepzibah Rani Gidla, Dr. Y. Kalyan Chakravarthy, Dr. Pavan Kumar Yanamadala
Aditya Pharmacy College, Aditya University, Surampalem, Andhra Pradesh, India

Abstract

Heart transplantation has emerged as a crucial intervention for patients suffering from end-stage heart failure, yet it is accompanied by considerable perioperative challenges. This review explores the essential anesthetic considerations associated with heart transplantation, a procedure characterized by the necessity for swift coordination, intricate patient management, and the presence of high-risk intraoperative scenarios. The role of cardiac anesthesiologists is vital in enhancing patient outcomes, beginning with a thorough preoperative evaluation that encompasses cardiovascular, pulmonary, renal, and hepatic assessments, as well as an appraisal of the patient's psychological preparedness. Anesthetic approaches must be customized to mitigate the risks of immunosuppressive complications, vascular damage, and infections, particularly in light of the immunocompromised status that follows transplantation. Innovations such as extracorporeal membrane oxygenation (ECMO) play a significant role in supporting cardiac function in complex cases, including those involving mechanical assist devices before transplantation. The postoperative period focuses on preventing organ rejection and infection, facilitating a gradual reduction in mechanical support, and ensuring sufficient pain management. The initiatives by win-india highlight the importance of integrated healthcare systems in advancing transplant practices..

Keywords: *Heart Transplantation, Anesthesia Management, Cardiac Anesthesia, Perioperative Care, Extracorporeal Membrane Oxygenation (ECMO), Ventricular Support*

Presented as Poster

AI In Drug Delivery And Development

Scan to View online

Presented by
M.Meenakshi ,T.Neha Sri, S.Pujitha
Sri Vasavi Institute of Pharmaceutical Sciences, Pedatadepalli, Andhra Pradesh, India

Abstract

Artificial intelligence (AI) has emerged as a powerful tool to revolutionize the healthcare sector, including drug delivery and development. It explores the current and future applications of AI in the pharmaceutical industry, focusing on drug delivery and development. It has various aspects such as smart drug delivery networks, drug repurposing, statistical modeling, and simulation of biotechnological and biological systems. In this the integration of AI with nanotechnologies and nanomedicines is also examined. AI mainly offers significant advancements in drug discovery by efficiently identifying compounds, validating drug targets, streamlining drug structures, and prioritizing response templates. Techniques like data mining, multitask learning, and high-throughput screening contribute to better drug discovery and development innovations. This also includes AI applications in drug formulation and delivery, clinical trials, drug safety, and pharmacovigilance. It addresses regulatory considerations and challenges associated with AI in pharmaceuticals, including privacy, data security, and interpretability of AI models. The review concludes with future perspectives, highlighting emerging trends, addressing limitations and biases in AI models, and emphasizing the importance of collaboration and knowledge sharing. It provides a comprehensive overview of AI's potential to transform the pharmaceutical industry and improve patient care while identifying further research and development areas.

Keywords: *Nano technology, Nano medicine,data security,drug safety, health care sector.*

Presented as Poster

A Novel Drug In Manufacturing Of Multi Layered Tablets

Scan to View online

Presented by
Pentakota Sandhya , Nalli Likhitha, Yerusu Deepika
Raghu College of Pharmacy,
Bheemunipatnam, Andhra Pradesh, India

Abstract

Multi layered tablets are combination of two or more active pharmaceutical ingredients for an improved therapeutic effect or to achieve a specific drug release profile. In multi layered tablet two or more active pharmaceutical ingredients can be combined where one layer or one drug may be for immediate release and the other layer of drug may be for sustained release of drug i.e., one layer is a loading dose and the other layer may be a maintenance dose. Multi layered tablets can help to overcome the drug interactions, the disadvantages of non-linearity associated with diffusion-controlled matrix devices providing an increased surface area resulting in an increased drug release rate with time. This abstract discusses the various kinetic models in multilayered tablets as well as the different techniques involved in the preparation of multi layered tablets.

Keywords: *Multilayered tablets, Immediate release, Controlled release, Drug loading*

Presented as Poster

Impurity Profiling In Pharmaceuticals

Scan to View online

Presented by
P. Vaishnavi, V. Sravya, S. Kavya
Raghu College of Pharmacy,
Bheemunipatnam, Andhra Pradesh, India

Abstract

The process of acquiring and evaluating data that establishes the biological safety of an individual purity in a pharmaceutical product. It involves identification, structure elucidation, quantitative determination of impurities and degradation products and bulk drugs materials and pharmaceutical formulations. It helps to ensure quality, efficacy and safety of drugs. Guidelines for impurity profiling are Q3A(R2) refers to the impurities in the new drug substance, Q3B(R2) refers to the impurity in new drug products, Q3C(R4) refers to the impurities from residual solvents. Sources of impurities includes organic, inorganic and residual solvents. Organic impurities are derived from plants, animals and human waste. Inorganic impurities often derived from the manufacturing process. The impurities are often reagents, ligands, catalysts, heavy metals and inorganic salts. Residual solvents are defined as organic volatile chemicals used in the manufacturing of drugs substance or excipients. Different analytical methods of impurity profiling are spectroscopic techniques which includes UV-VIS, IR, NMR ,Mass etc. and chromatographic techniques including column ,TLC ,HPTLC ,HPLC ,UPLC ,GC ,SFC. Whereas Hyphenated techniques include LC-MS, GC-MS, LC-IR ,LC-NMR.

Keywords:

Presented as Poster

Polycystic Ovarian Syndrome

Scan to View online

Presented by
A.Anusha T.Bindu Kalyani A.Varsha Sai Sri
VJ's College of Pharmacy, Rajahmundry, Andhra Pradesh, India

Abstract

Polycystc ovary syndrome (PCOS) is a widespread reproductve disorder that encompasses many associated health conditons and has an impact on various metabolic processes. PCOS is depicted by hyperandrogenism, polycystc ovaries, and anovulaton. It increases the risk of insulin resistance (IR), type 2 diabetes, obesity, and cardiovascular disease. The etology of the disease remains unclear, and the subjectve phenotype makes a united diagnosis difcult among physicians. It seems to be a familial genetc syndrome caused by a combinaton of environmental and genetc factors. It can be linked with metabolic disorders in frst-degree family members. PCOS is the cause of up to 30% of infertlity in couples seeking treatment. Currently, thereis no cure for PCOS. Despite the growing incidence of this syndrome, limited research has been done that encompasses the entrety of PCOS spectrum. In this review, the current status and possible future perspectve will be discussed.

***Keywords**: Polycystc ovary syndrome, PCOS, Obesity, Insulin Resistance, Diabetes, Metormin*

Presented as Poster

An Alarming Issues In Food Poisoning: A Brief Study

Scan to View online

Presented by
Rohmit Singh, Mohd Waseem, Bilal Majeed Dar, Kanan Sharma, Abibe Kumar
School of Pharmaceutical Sciences & Technologies, JNTU, Kakinada, Andhra Pradesh, India

Abstract

Food poisoning is an acute illness, usually of sudden onset, brought about by eating contaminated or poisonous food. The symptoms normally include abdominal pain, diarrhoea, nausea, vomiting and fever. Food poisoning, also known as foodborne illness, occurs when you consume contaminated food or beverages. It's typically caused by infectious organisms—such as bacteria, viruses, and parasites—or their toxins. Symptoms can appear within hours of consuming contaminated food or may take days or even weeks to manifest. Food poisoning typically concludes with symptom resolution, hydration, and a gradual return to normal eating, although severe cases may need medical intervention. A case-control study was conducted. Patients either symptomatic of food poisoning (cases) or asymptomatic (controls) eating at the hospital cafeteria were included. To identify the source of the outbreak, sanitary control factors were assessed. Microbiological studies and the mast cell tryptase test were performed. Food poisoning after the consumption of fish from the family Scombridae is the most common food poisoning involving fish worldwide and it includes fish commonly consumed such as tuna, herring, sardines, anchovies, mackerel and bonito. The poisoning occurs by the ingestion of fish contaminated by histamine. The usual clinical presentation is an allergic reaction that appears between a few minutes and a few hours after ingestion.

Keywords: *Food poisoning, illness issues, the symptoms, the case publications, the issues of food poisoning occurs due to scombroids.*

Presented as Poster

Virtual Laboratories Digital Simulation Of Physical Labs.

Scan to View online

Presented by
Y.Yasodha,K.Naga Chandrika,K.Usharani
Viswanadha Institute of Pharmaceutical Sciences, Sontyam, Visakhapatnam, Andhra Pradesh, India

Abstract

Virtual laboratories are digital platforms that simulate real-world laboratory environments, allowing users to perform experiments and practice scientific techniques without physical resources. This study explores the impact and efficacy of virtual laboratories in educational settings, particularly in science and engineering disciplines. Virtual laboratories offer flexible, safe, and cost-effective solutions for students, enabling experimental learning through interactive simulations and real-time feedback. Making quality education more accessible as educational institutions increasingly adopt digital tools, virtual laboratories represent a powerful resource for supplementing traditional lab experiences and meeting diverse learner needs. Virtual laboratories are transforming science and engineering education by providing students with immersive lab experiences accessible from any location. Through high-fidelity simulations, virtual laboratories enable learners to conduct experiments, test hypotheses, and develop technical skills without the limitations of physical lab space. Our findings suggest that virtual laboratories not only complement traditional labs but also foster critical thinking and adaptability in students, preparing them for real-world scientific and engineering challenges. Increased communication between students on the internet helps with the exchange of ideas and experiences.

Keywords: *Keywords: virtual laboratories, digital simulations, cost effective solutions, technical skill development, hypotheses testing*

Presented as Poster

Silver Nano Particles Using Vernonia Amygdalina

Scan to View online

Presented by
B.V.Varshitha, K. Kavitha , K. Siddardha, B.Mohan
Raghu College of Pharmacy,
Bheemunipatnam, Andhra Pradesh, India

Abstract

The green nanoparticles synthesis method from leaves extract revealed full an economical, sustainable and eco-friendly method. In this study, the leaf extract of Vernonia amygdalina was as a reducing and capping agent for the synthesis of silver nanoparticles (AgNPs). M/DW binary solvent was selected for its relatively better extraction performance than methanol, ethanol, distilled water and ethanol/distilled water. Furthermore, the effect of solvent ratio of M/DW, precursor concentration, ratio of silver nitrate (AgNO) to plant extract, temperature, time and pH on the synthesis of AgNPs was carried out. Greenly synthesized Agents was confirmed using UV-Vis spectroscopy and characterized by XRD and FT-IR. Besides, its antimicrobial activities were also evaluated using agar diffusion techniques. The UV-Vis spectra showed specific Surface Plasmon Resonance (SPR) absorption peaks between 411 nm and 430 nm which revealed the formation of AgNPs during the synthesis. The nanoparticle synthesis was further confirmed by XRD analysis. Phytochemical screening test and FT-IR analysis of V. amygdalina leaves extract revealed the existence of phenolic, Tannin, saponins and flavonoid groups, which capped the nanoparticles during the synthesis. The antibacterial activities of the synthesized AgNPs were evaluated against Gram-positive bacteria (S. pyogenes and S. aureus) and Gram-negative bacteria
(E. coli and P. aeruginosa) and higher inhibition zones were observed.

Keywords: *Nano particles, Vernonia amygdalina, UV spectroscopy, XRD analysis, Anti bacterial*

Presented as Poster

Variations In Breast Cancer - An Overview

Scan to View online

Presented by
S.Baby Rani, G. Sanjana
VJ's College of Pharmacy, Rajahmundry, Andhra Pradesh, India

Abstract

Breast cancer ranked as 2nd predominant malignancy that is affecting women worldwide. It is a Heterogeneous cancer, encompasses multiple Subtypes with distinct molecular, Histological & clinical characteristics. An accurate classification is crucial for tailored treatment strategies & improved patient outcomes. Some of them are DCIS, IDC, ILC, Paget's disease, phyllodes tumor. Breast cancer is accounts for 25-30% of all cancer Cases in India. Approximately 1.5 lack new cases are diagnosed annually. Breast cancer incidence rate in India is 28.25.8/100,000 women. In India 12-15, of cancer deaths are accounted, nearly 90,000 women die from Breast cancer annually mortality rate is 12.5/100,000, at early state 20-30% of cases can be detected. This review explores about the pathophysiology, types and treatment of breast cancer.

Keywords: *DCIS, IDC, ILC, Mucin, HER 2 +VE, Mamogram, IBC, Mastocarcinoma*

Presented as Poster

Increased Anti Biotic Resistance Due To Self Medication

Scan to View online

Presented by
P. Grace Sowmya , M.Chandra Lekha,
S.Usha Rani, P.V.S.S. Pravallika
Raghu College of Pharmacy,
Bheemunipatnam, Andhra Pradesh, India

Abstract

The present study aims to explore the crisis of antibiotic resistance and discover more about the current challenges related to self-medication. The current challenges related to antibiotic resistance are unique and differ from the challenges of the past since new bacterial pathogens are involved and continue to evolve. Antibiotic resistance can be reduced by using antibiotics prudently based on guidelines of antimicrobial stewardship programs (ASPs) and various data such as pharmacokinetic (PK) and pharmacodynamic (PD) properties of antibiotics, diagnostic testing, antimicrobial susceptibility testing (AST), clinical response, and effects on the micro biota, as well as by new antibiotic developments. The controlled use of antibiotics in food animals is another cornerstone among efforts to reduce antibiotic resistance. The problem of antibiotic resistance can be minimized only by concerted efforts of all members of society for ensuring the continued efficiency of antibiotics.Antibiotic resistance is one of the biggest threats to global health, food security, and development today. A growing number of infections such as pneumonia, tuberculosis, gonorrhoea, and salmonellosis are becoming harder to treat as the antibiotics used to treat them become less effective. Antibiotic resistance leads to longer hospital stays, higher medical costs and increased mortality.

Keywords: *Antibiotic resistance, strategy, antibiotic prescribing, antibiotic stewardship programs, education, hygiene, new antibiotics*

Presented as Poster

Innovative Niosome Drug Delivery:Unlocking Potent Antihelmentic Effects From Nature

Scan to View online

Presented by
G.Ramkarishna, K.Iswarya, B. Sailakshmi, A.Kavitha, Ch Jahnavi
Aditya Pharmacy College, Aditya University, Surampalem, Andhra Pradesh, India

Abstract

The theory on andrographis paniculata, a member of the acanthaceae family, explores its chemical composition, extraction methods, and potential as a drug delivery system using niosomes. It contains various compounds such as polyphenols, flavonoids, diterpenes, alkaloids, and key components like andrographolide. The extraction process involves ethanol pre-extraction followed by fractionation. Niosomes, a novel drug delivery system, are formulated using andrographis paniculata, tween 80, span 80, cholesterol, and chloroform. The process includes mixing ingredients, evaporating chloroform, and forming niosomes through sonication and centrifugation. Characterization techniques like ir spectroscopy confirm the presence of polyphenols. Percentage entrapment efficiency is determined to be 83.7%, indicating effective drug encapsulation. *In vivo* characterization compares the anthelmintic activity of andrographis paniculata with albendazole, a standard drug, showing promising results in paralyzing and killing earthworms. The discussion highlights the superior action of andrographis paniculata compared to the marketed drug, indicating its potential as an anthelmintic agent. This study suggests that andrographis paniculata holds promise for addressing parasitic infections due to its potent anthelmintic activity. Further research and application of this natural compound could lead to the development of effective treatments for parasitic infections in the future.

Keywords: *Andrographis Paniculata, Niosomes, Drug Delivery System, Anthelmintic Activity, Andrographolide, Extraction*

Presented as Poster

Zebrafish-An Animal Model For Biomedical Research

Scan to View online

Presented by
S .Poojitha, N.Jaya Sri, Y. Sailaja
VV Institute of Pharmaceutical Sciences,
Gudlavalleru, Andhra Pradesh, India

Abstract

Compared to other vertebrate models for disease modeling, zebrafish have several advantages for large-scale genetic mutant and therapeutic compound screenings, among others, for biomedical research applications. The impactful developments of CRISPR and next-generation sequencing technology are further accelerating the understanding of the molecular mechanisms of human genetic diseases through disease modeling in zebrafish. It is within these efforts that hope for the future of precision medicine resides: new diagnostic and therapeutic approaches are provided. This review especially summarizes disease models in zebrafish for biomedical research on developmental disorders, mental disorders, and metabolic diseases.

Keywords: *Human hereditary disease, developmental disorder, next sequential, zebrafish*

Presented as Poster

Development Of Sustained - Release Rimegepant Tablets Using Jackfruit Seed Starch As A Natural Polymer.

Scan to View online

Presented by
Nagireddy Gayatri Satya Devi, Sadhu Rakesh, Sarakula Keerthi, Sayyad Rahimunnisa
Aditya Pharmacy College, Aditya University, Surampalem, Andhra Pradesh, India

Abstract

The purpose of this work was to assess the use of jackfruit seed starch as a natural polymer in developing sustained-release tablets of rimegepant, a new calcitonin gene-related peptide (cgrp) receptor antagonist for migraine treatment. Jackfruit seed starch was extracted, characterized, and incorporated into the tablet matrix at concentrations of 10%, 15%, and 20%. The goal was to evaluate the polymer's effectiveness in modulating the release of rimegepant over a 12-hour period. Tablets containing 20% jackfruit seed starch demonstrated optimal sustained-release profiles, with a prolonged and controlled drug release. The study concludes that jackfruit seed starch can be a viable natural alternative to synthetic polymers in sustained-release drug delivery systems.

Keywords: *Rimegepant, Sustained -Release, Jackfruit Seed Starch , Natural Polymer,Drug Delivery.*

Presented as Poster

A Modern Manufacturing System Facilitates Pharmaceutical Operations

Scan to View online

Presented by
Yegi Sirisha, Yerra Pallavi, Varri Ambica Taruni
Aditya Pharmacy College, Aditya University, Surampalem, Andhra Pradesh, India

Abstract

The "lean manufacturing" ideology in pharmaceutical operations is primarily concerned with reducing or eliminating waste and increasing production with enhanced safety and efficacy. By implementing the four important lean principles like value stream mapping, just in time production, 5s, kaizen, and maintenance and total production. Initially value stream mapping enhances the production process by identifying and removing waste; just-in-time production focuses on promoting a lower-cost supply chain in increased demand situations; and 5s and kaizen are tools that organizes the workspace safe and clean to workspace while also encourages step-by-step continuous improvement. Higher output with fewer resources can be achieved through lean manufacturing's ability to increase productivity and may enhance customer satisfaction by meeting customer expectations and delivering items on schedule. Costs like labor, energy, and raw material utilization can be considerably decreased by getting rid of waste and increasing efficiency. Despite the many advantages of lean manufacturing, it's important to recognize some of its possible disadvantages, including initial investment, supply chain dependence, resistance to new change, lack of flexibility, and greater workload. Companies must carefully address these issues and adopt a progressive transformation strategy in order to get success using the lean manufacturing strategies.

***Keywords*::** *production,waste, 5S, Kaizen, supply chain, value stream mapping,*

Presented as Poster

Epidermodysplasia Verruciformis (Tree Man Syndrome): A Rare Genetic Disorder

Scan to View online

Presented by
B. Surekha, S. Sushma
VJ's College of Pharmacy, Rajahmundry, Andhra Pradesh, India

Abstract

Epidermodysplasia Verruciformis (EV), also known as Tree Man Syndrome, is an extremely rare genetic disorder characterized by an abnormal susceptibility to human papillomavirus (HPV) infections. This condition leads to the growth of multiple wart-like lesions on the skin, which can resemble tree bark. EV is inherited in an autosomal recessive pattern and is associated with mutations in the EVER1 and EVER2 genes. Uncontrolled infections result in the growth of scaly macules and papules similar to tree bark, mainly on the hands and feet. Patients here with slightly scaly, flat, red-brown macules on the neck, face and body, chronic particularly around the penial area, seborrheic keratosis-like lesions or verruca-like papillomatous lesions, and pinkish-red plane papules on the hands, upper and lower extremities, and face. Clinical diagnostic features are enduring eruptions of flat wart-like papules, pityriasis versicolor-like macules, cutaneous horn-like lesions, and development of cutaneous carcinomas. No curative treatment has been established yet. Epidermodysplasia Verruciforms (EV) is sometimes called tree-man disease or human tree disease. This condition was first identified in 1922 it is so rare that doctors can confirm 200 cases of it since them. EV is a genetic disorder that can't be predicted. There are no tests for human tree disease. The given article review about the Ethiology and Pathophysiology and diagnosis of the tree man syndrome.

Keywords: *Epidermodyplasia Verruciformis, Tree man syndrome, Human papillomavirus, Genetic Disorder, Skin Lesions, Immunodeficiency.*

Presented as Poster

Medication Adherence And Its Effect On Clinical Outcomes In Diabetic Patients

Scan to View online

Presented by
Anju. K. Abraham
Aditya College of Pharmacy, Aditya University, Surampalem, Andhra Pradesh, India

Abstract

In a secondary hospital, a prospective observational study lasting six months was conducted to evaluate the clinical results and adherence to oral hypoglycemic medicines in diabetic outpatients who were above the age of eighteen and of both genders. The study's focus was on the patients' glycemic level. Out of 90 patients with diabetes, 47.78% were male, 52.22% were female, 37.8% were between the ages of 61 and 70, and 63.31 were prescribed a combination of metformin and glibenclamide, whereas 22.2% were prescribed metformin monotherapy. This difference was directly correlated with the patients' mean medication possession ratio. Based on the medicine possession ratio value, it was found in this study that 83.3% of patients were not adhering to their treatment. The outcome also demonstrated a statistically significant variation in patient clinical outcomes according to drug compliance. In conclusion, establishing a correlation between medication adherence and quality of life in the diabetic community could be a useful strategy to maintain and enhance health outcomes.

Keywords: *Medication Adherence, Monotherapy, Drug Compliance*

Presented as Poster

In Silicon Modeling Computer Simulation Instead Of Biological Studies

Scan to View online

Presented by
Neha Kumari, P.N.S.Prasanna, P.Devi Thanuja, D.Sai Monisha.
Viswanadha Institute of Pharmaceutical Sciences, Sontyam, Visakhapatnam, Andhra Pradesh, India

Abstract

In silico modelling is a computational approach that utilizes computer simulations to study biological systems, from molecules to organisms. This method involves using virtual simulations to predict molecular properties, thereby reducing the need for expensive and time-consuming experiments. It provides a powerful tool for understanding complex biological processes, predicting the outcomes of interventions and accelerating drug discovery. Silicon modelling uses silicon as a base material to create detailed and accurate models that represent physical structures and systems, especially in fields such as electronics, nanotechnology, and material sciences. By combining computational and experimental methods, researchers can generate hypotheses that are testable through experimentation. The process includes encoding hypotheses about mechanisms of cellular function and disease pathogenesis, contributing to the identification of new drug targets. These models facilitate rapid advancements through high-throughput biological data. In recent developments, in silico models have enabled the creation of virtual tissues and organs, simulating complex physiological processes. In silico models complement, rather than replace, traditional experimental research, including *in vivo* models, animal testing, and clinical trials, making it a vital tool in modern scientific exploration.

Keywords: *Insilico modelling, virtual simulations, drug discovery, computational methods,hypotheses generation*

Presented as Poster

Formulation And Evaluation Of Lamivudine Loaded Microspheres

Scan to View online

Presented by
Malakar Vandana Rani
Vignan Institute of Pharmaceutical Technology, Visakhapatnam, Andhra Pradesh, India

Abstract

The main objective of the present work was to develop a formulation with increased therapeutic efficacy, reduced frequency of administration and improved patient compliance by developing sustained release microspheres of Lamivudine using different polymers to study its functionality for sustained release of drug from microspheres formulations. Different concentrations of polymers like sodium alginate, HPMC, sodium CMC, chitosan was selected for the study. Microspheres were prepared by using ionic- gelation method. Prepared microspheres were evaluated for particle size, flow properties, drug content, and entrapment efficiency. After evaluation of physical properties of microspheres, the *in-vitro* release study was performed in 0.1 N Hcl as buffer for 1 hr. after that replace with 6.8 phosphate buffer up to 8hrs. After 8 hrs. of study microspheres with sodium CMC showed maximum release (99.98%). Among all the formulations F7 which contain 200 mg of sodium CMC release the drug which follows first order kinetics. The FTIR study shows that there was no chemical interaction between drug and excipients.

Keywords: *Lamivudine, Sodium alginate, Hydroxy Propyl Methyl Cellulose, Sodium Carboxy Methyl Cellulose, Chitosan, Microspheres*

Presented as Poster

A Novel Therapeutic Approach Of Targeted Nucleic Acid Delivery System

Scan to View online

Presented by
Teki Swathi Revathi Naga Lakshmi,
Sarampati Vishnu Surya Kala
Aditya Pharmacy College, Aditya University, Surampalem, Andhra Pradesh, India

Abstract

Nucleic acid delivery system is a technique designed for efficient delivery of nucleic acids (dna, rna) into cells to modify gene expression, treat genetic diseases or provide therapeutic benefits." Enhancement of gene therapy efficacy is done by developing targeted nanoparticles for nucleic acid delivery to view the advancements and challenges in gene therapy. Nucleic acids are the macromolecules which are used to carry information in cells, and also useful to makeup genetic material. Nucleic acid delivery systems are mainly based on two types of delivery systems they are, viral based delivery system and non-viral delivery system. Viral vectors mainly include retrovirus, adenovirus, adeno associated vectors. Non- viral delivery systems includes liposome delivery, nanoparticle delivery, electroporation, microinjection, gene gun. Gene therapy results in enhanced gene expression mechanism, targeted nanoparticles increased specificity, estimated delivery efficacy in invitro and invivo therapy system. Gene therapy will be very useful for the prevention of those diseases for future generations. "gene therapy is highly promising for clinical applications involving the insertion of a functioning nucleic acid into dysfunctioning cells to provide correct cellular function." Targeted nucleic acid delivery system holds potentiality for treating genetic diseases. Efficient delivery of nucleic acids is crucial for gene therapies success. Nucleic acid based therapeutic delivery system is the technique of gene therapy useful for treatment of many genetic disorders.

Keywords: *Gene therapy, nucleic acid delivery, precision medicine, targeted delivery and nanoparticles, vector based delivery.*

Presented as Poster

Self Medication - A Current Challenge

Scan to View online

Presented by
D.Charishma,K.Sridevi B.Lasya
VJ's College of Pharmacy, Rajahmundry,
Andhra Pradesh, India

Abstract

Self-medication is a global phenomenon and potential contributor to human pathogen resistance to antibiotics. The adverse consequences of such practices should always be emphasized to the community and steps to curb it. Rampant irrational use of antimicrobials without medical guidance may result in greater probability of inappropriate, incorrect, or undue therapy, missed diagnosis, delays in appropriate treatment, pathogen resistance and increased morbidity. This review focused on the self-medication of allopathic drugs, their use, its safety and reason for using it. It would be safe, if the people who are using it, have sufficient knowledge about its dose, time of intake, side effect on over dose, but due to lack of information it can cause serious effects such as antibiotic resistance, skin problem, hypersensitivity and allergy. There is need to augment awareness and implement legislations to promote judicious and safe practices. Improved knowledge and understanding about self-medication may result in rationale use and thus limit emerging microbial resistance issues. Articles which were published in peer reviewed journals, World Self-Medication Industry and World Health Organization websites relating to self-medication reviewed.

Keywords: *Allopathic drugs, antibiotic resistance, self-medication*

Presented as Poster

Overview Of Opioid Epidemic

Scan to View online

Presented by
Sai Kiran , Amulya , Gowri Tejaswani, Bhavana
School of Pharmaceutical Sciences & Technologies, JNTU, Kakinada, Andhra Pradesh, India

Abstract

Opioid Addiction in the United State has come to national attention as Opioid overdose related deaths have risen at alarming rates. Overcoming opioid epidemic becomes a high priority for not only government but also health care providers. In this Poster, we present our work on effects opioid on present situation particularly on Pregnant Women, Opioid crises related to AI (ARTIFICIAL INTELLIGENCE) based on the history of patients in Opioid Epidemic in Resource center. In our poster presentation, we are presenting that- National Overdose deaths involving any Opioid among all ages, by Sex (1999-2022). We are representing our criteria (Opioid Overdose) in World Map at present situation. It also includes Education and Awareness towards Opioid Epidemic. It ensures to improve the prescription practice. The Higher the Opioid dose the higher the risk for misuse and overdose steps. Prolonged duration, prolonged use is associated with significant risk of addiction. Opioid mortality prevalence is higher in people who are middle-aged and have substance abuse and Psychiatric comorbidities. Risk assessment and prevention include knowledge of patient factors that may contribute to misuse, abuse, addiction, suicide and respiratory depression

Keywords: *Opioid, artificial intelligence, respiratory depression, risk assessment, psychiatric comorbidities*

Presented as Poster

The Future Of Pharmacy: How Telemedicine And Digital Health Are Changing The Field

Scan to View online

Presented by
Dhanusri Bhupathi
Aditya Pharmacy College, Aditya University, Surampalem, Andhra Pradesh, India

Abstract

The future of pharmacy is changing fastly due to telemedicine and digital health. Telemedicine permits people to talk with doctors from home by using video calls or apps, so they don't routinely have to visit the hospital or clinic. This is modifying how pharmacies work too. More patients now get their prescriptions and guided from pharmacists on online. Pharmacists have an major role in this new way of healthcare. They help make sure patients are taking the right medications, even when consultations are done indirectly. Digital devices, like health apps and electronic prescriptions, permits the pharmacists to keep track of patients' medication history and help them continue their treatment plans. This makes it easier to detect the problems easily and avoid mistakes, which makes patients healthier. Telepharmacy is also extremely well known . This also permits pharmacists to give guidance through video chats, which is mainly useful for the people who live afar from a pharmacy. Digital health also makes it simpler for pharmacists, doctors, and other healthcare workers to work together, so patients get improved overall care. As technology keeps going , pharmacists will proceed to take on major roles in digital healthcare. They are using new equipments to help patients handle their medications better and improve health services for everyone. Telemedicine and digital health are making healthcare easier to approch and more useful for people everywhere.

Keywords: *Telemedicine, Digital health, pharmacist, electronic prescription , Health apps.,*

Presented as Poster

Study On Ayurvedic Formulation- Madhumeha Churnam In The Treatment Of Diabetes.

Scan to View online

Presented by
Dr. K. Ravi Shankar, K. Gnaneswari, Dr. N Divya.
Aditya College of Pharmacy, Aditya University, Surampalem, Andhra Pradesh, India

Abstract

The indigenous ayurvedic formulation, madhumeha churnam is taken up to evaluate its hypoglycemic and hypolipidemic activities. Several traditional medicinal plants parts like gymnema sylvestre, andrographis paniculata, senna alexandrina, azadirachta indica, zingiber officinale, murraya koenigii, were used and an ayurvedic formulation is prepared to explore the therapeutic potential. Diabetes is induced to rats using alloxan monohydrate and these diabetic rats were selected for the research study. The effect of this formulation on lipid profile is also estimated and the results obtained were tabulated and compared with the standard drug glibenclamide.

Keywords: *Madhumeha Churnam, Hypoglycemic, Hypolipidemic, Alloxan, Standard Drug Glibenclamide.*

Presented as Poster

Comparision Of Vesicular Carriers

Scan to View online

Presented by
D.Suchitra, K.Syamala, G.Tejasree,
D.Nikhila Reddy
Raghu College of Pharmacy,
Bheemunipatnam, Andhra Pradesh, India

Abstract

Now a days people want advanced technologies to meet their pharmaceutical demands like increased bioavailability or increased therapeutic effects etc. In that view scientist have introduced various vesicular carriers so called as novel drug delivery systems. Novel Drug delivery System (NDDS) refers to the approaches, formulations, technologies, and systems for transporting a pharmaceutical compound in the body as needed to safely achieve its desired therapeutic effects. It may involve scientific site-targeting within the body, or it might involve facilitating systemic pharmacokinetics; in any case, it is typically concerned with both quantity and duration of drug presence. The are fluctuation of drug level in blood depending upon dosage form. Therefore to maintain the drug concentration within therapeutically effective range need novel drug delivery system. There are several factors like temperature, cost, drug solubility which are effecting the vesicular carriers in drug delivery systems. Basically the basic mechanism of vesicular carriers is the drug is encapsulated in the internal core. The drugs are dissolved in the internal core both hydrophobic and hydrophilic drugs. When the carriers come in contact with membrane of the targeted organ, the drug content is released. Novel cosmetic delivery systems reviewed here possess enormous potential as next-generation smarter carrier systems.

Keywords: *Carriers, dosage forms, encapsulation, hydrophobic, hydrophilic, liposomes, phytosomes*

Presented as Poster

Enhanced Dissolution Of Ritonavir Through Solid Dispersion With Synergistic Carriers : A Novel Formulation Approach

Scan to View online

Presented by
Thummala Udaya Kumar, Adapa Vijay Mounika
Aditya Pharmacy College, Aditya University, Surampalem, Andhra Pradesh, India

Abstract

The primary aim of this study was to enhance the dissolution rate of ritonavir, a poorly water-soluble drug, by formulating solid dispersions with various carriers to improve its bioavailability. A novel approach was employed using a four-component mixture of pvp, sls, mannitol, and urea in different ratios. The solvent evaporation method was used to prepare solid dispersions of ritonavir with drug-carrier ratios of 1:2 and 1:4. The formulations were then evaluated for *In vivo* dissolution using usp apparatus ii. Among the formulations, F13, containing a 1:4 ratio of ritonavir and the carrier mixture, achieved the highest dissolution rate of 98.09% within 60 minutes. This represented a 3.32-fold increase compared to the marketed product and a 1.31-fold increase compared to pure ritonavir (F1). The findings highlight that the combination of carriers used in F13 significantly enhanced the dissolution rate of ritonavir. This formulation approach provides a promising solution to improve ritonavir's bioavailability and has the potential for patenting and commercialization.

Keywords: *Dissolution Rate ,Solvent Evaporation Method ,Bioavailability*

Presented as Poster

Computational Advancements In Detection Of Multidrug Resistance

Scan to View online

Presented by
Jagarlamudi Tanuja Bhagyasri
Chalapathi Institute of Pharmaceutical Sciences, Lam, Andhra Pradesh, India

Abstract

Antibiotics are chemical substances that are used to treat a variety of infections caused by microbes , overtimes due to irrational usage ,drug misuse, lack of strong regulatory measures has accelerated the antimicrobial resistance due to development of antimicrobial resistant genes . Antibiotic resistance is a global problem threatening the modern world, According to the Global Antimicrobial Resistance Surveillance System report in 2017, the major clinically relevant antibiotic resistance species are Escherichia coli, Klebsiella pneumoniae, Acinetobacter species, Staphylococcusaureus, Salmonella species,Shigella species., Streptococcus pneumoniae, and Neisseria gonorrhoeae. They acquire drug resistance by development of efflux pumps,target modification, enzymatic bypass ,target mimicry and several other strategies. To decelerate the spread of antibiotic resistant genes, surveillance of the resistome is of prior importance. Therefore, in this review we discuss about combating antimicrobial resistance by applications of whole-genome sequencing and metagenomics together with machine learning models for survelliance of resistosomes .

Keywords: *Resistosome, whole genome sequencing, metagenomics, multidrug resistance, resistant genes*

Presented as Poster

Formulation Of Tafamidis Immediate-Release Tablets Using Okra Gum As A Natural Disintegrant

Scan to View online

Presented by
Udaya Kumar Thummala, Chunduri Harshini, Dodda Likhitha
Aditya Pharmacy College, Aditya University, Surampalem, Andhra Pradesh, India

Abstract

The purpose of this research was to investigate the use of okra gum as a natural disintegrant in the formulation of immediate-release tafamidis tablets. Okra gum was extracted, processed, and incorporated into tablet formulations at concentrations of 5%, 10%, and 15% through direct compression. The study assessed disintegration time, friability, and tablet hardness. Results indicated that the 10% okra gum formulation provided rapid disintegration and met pharmacopoeial standards for tablet strength. The research showed that okra gum could be a promising natural disintegrant for immediate-release formulations, providing a viable alternative to synthetic excipients.

Keywords: *Tafamidis, Okra Gum, Natural Disintegrant, Immediate-Release, Tablet Formulation.*

Presented as Poster

Molecular Dynamics Simulations

Scan to View online

Presented by
Vanitha,Swetha,Avinash,Sharma
Viswanadha Institute of Pharmaceutical Sciences, Sontyam, Visakhapatnam, Andhra Pradesh, India

Abstract

Molecular dynamics is seriously cool stuff! It's all about simulating the movements of particles in biological macromolecules, giving us the lowdown on how atoms in proteins or DNA jiggle around over time. This knowledge is like a secret weapon, helping us understand things like how flexibility affects binding to molecules and how quickly photosynthesis can soak up that electron transfer state. And get this - molecular dynamics is even helping us figure out protein structures from NMR, refine X-ray crystal structures faster than ever, and calculate the energy changes when proteins mutate MDAnalysis is a fantastic library for conducting structural and temporal analysis of molecular dynamics (MD) simulation trajectories and individual protein structures. It's built in Python with some performance-critical code in C, making it super fast. The library leverages the NumPy package to present trajectory data as efficient NumPy arrays, delivering incredible performance even on systems with millions of particles. MDAnalysis supports various file formats from simulation packages like CHARMM, Gromacs, Amber, NAMD, and the Protein Data Bank format. What's more, it allows for atom selection using a syntax similar to CHARMM's powerful selection commands. Whether you're a novice or experienced programmer, MDAnalysis empowers you to quickly develop your own analytical tools and access trajectory data in an easily accessible manner, making interactive explorative analysis a breeze. It's been tested on most Unix-based platforms such as Linux and Mac OS X, ensuring its reliability and effectiveness.

Keywords:

Presented as Poster

Isolation Of Microorganisms From Detoreiated Banaana

Scan to View online

Presented by

Seetha Maha Lakshmi Vakkapatla, Pravallika . V

School of Pharmaceutical Sciences & Technologies, JNTU, Kakinada, Andhra Pradesh, India

Abstract

This project work was carried out to isolate and identify the microorganism involved in the spoilage of banana fruit (Musa acuminata) sold in some selected markets in kakinada. Microorganisms associated with spoilage of banana (Musa acuminata) were studied using standard microbiological methods. The serial dilution method was employed using nutrient agar. The microorganisms detected are staphylococcus spp majorly along with Other microorganisms.The bacterial loads were high enough to cause food spoilage or food infection. The presence of the isolates may be due to improper hygienic practices from the point of harvesting, transportation and storage by handlers. Above all, the high moisture content of banana fruit (Musa acuminata) makes it highly perishable as its supports the growth of microorganisms.

Keywords: *Microorganisms, spoilage, banana*

Presented as Poster

Xenoestrogen Preventable Causes Of Breast Cancer

Scan to View online

Presented by
P Deepika, K.Suma Sarvani, P Rupasree, K Tejarani
VJ's College of Pharmacy, Rajahmundry, Andhra Pradesh, India

Abstract

Changes in documented risk factors for breast cancer and rates of screening cannot completely explain recent increases in incidence or mortality. Established risk factors for breast cancer, including genetics, account for at best 30% of cases. Most of these risk factors can be linked to total lifetime exposure to bioavailable estrogens. Experimental evidence reveals that compounds such as some chlorinated organics, polycyclic aromatic hydrocarbons (PAHs), triazine herbicides, and pharmaceuticals affect estrogen production and metabolism and thus function as xenoestrogens. As the proportion of inherited breast cancer in the population is small, most breast cancers are due to acquired mutations. Thus, the induction of breast cancer in the majority of cases stems from interactions between host factors, including genetics and environmental carcinogens. series of major epidemiologic studies need to be developed to evaluate this hypothesis, including studies of estrogen metabolism, the role of specific xenoestrogenic substances in breast cancer, and relevant genetic-environmental interactions. In addition, experimental studies are needed to evaluate biologic markers of suspect xenoestrogens and biologic markers of host susceptibility and identify pathways of estrogenicity that affect the development of breast cancer. If xenoestrogens do play a role in breast cancer, reductions in exposure will provide an opportunity for primary prevention of this growing disease.

Keywords: *Breast Cancer , Polycyclic Aromatic Hydrocarbans , Xenoestrogenic Compound , Acquired Inhertence*

Presented as Poster

Quinazoline Derivatives: Recent Structure With Potential Antibacterial, Antituberculosis Activities.

Scan to View online

Presented by
V.Harini Tejasri,B.Suchitra,P.Supriya
Aditya Pharmacy College, Aditya University,
Surampalem, Andhra Pradesh, India

Abstract

In recent years, the overuse of antibiotics has resulted in the emergence of antibiotic resistance, which is a serious global health problem. Methicillin-resistant staphylococcus aureus (mrsa) is a common and virulent bacterium in clinical practice. Numerous researchers have focused on developing new candidate drugs that are effective, less toxic, and can overcome mrsa resistance. Thiazole derivatives have been found to exhibit antibacterial activity against drug-sensitive and drug-resistant pathogens. By hybridizing thiazole with other antibacterial pharmacophores, it is possible to obtain more effective antibacterial candidate drugs. Thiazole derivatives have shown potential in developing new drugs that can overcome drug resistance, reduce toxicity, and improve pharmacokinetic characteristics. This article reviews the recent progress of thiazole compounds as potential antibacterial compounds and examines the structure-activity relationship (sar) in various directions. It covers articles published from 2018 to 2023, providing a comprehensive platform to plan and develop new thiazole-based small mrsa growth inhibitors with minimal side effects.

Keywords: *Mrsa,Sar,Thiazole Derivatives, New Thiazole Based Small Mrsa Growth Inhibitors,Pharmacokinetics.*

Presented as Poster

Aquaculture Derived Hybrid Skin Patches For Wound Healing

Scan to View online

Presented by
Mohammad Johaparvaz, Pusala Durga Varalaxmi, Marukuthi Satya Bhavani, Adapa Tejaswini Bhargavi
VJ's College of Pharmacy, Rajahmundry, Andhra Pradesh, India

Abstract

ABSTRACT:
Natural biomaterials have been widely applied in wound treatment. Hotspots in this area are focused on reducing their immunogenicity and improving their therapeutic effect. In this work, we present a novel aquaculture derived hybrid skin patch based on Acellular Fish Skin (AFS) and Chitosan (CS) for wound healing. Such functional patch was simply constructed by infiltrating the Vascular Endothelial Growth Factor (VEGF)-loaded CS pregel into the porous scaffold of the AFS. As the natural molecules and structure of fish skin are well-retained during the synthesis processes, the final patch presented brilliant tensile property, water-absorption property, good bio-compatibility and low immunogenicity. In addition, the integrated CS and VEGF endow the patch with antibacterial and angiogenesis capability respectively for promoting tissue growth and wound healing. Thus, in a full-thickness wound rat model, the hybrid patch has been demonstrated with dramatic therapeutic efficacy in inhibiting inflammatory, accelerating angiogenesis, collagen deposition, and tissue generation during the wound repair procedure. These features imply the practical value of this multifunctional aquaculture derived hybrid skin patch in clinical wound management.

Keywords: *Wound Healing, Patch, Fish Skin, Bioactive, Biomaterial*

Presented as Poster

Pharmacogenomics Predectives

Scan to View online

Presented by
Chelle Amrutha Varshini, Yanamandra Sridevi
School of Pharmaceutical Sciences & Technologies, JNTU, Kakinada, Andhra Pradesh, India

Abstract

Pharmacogenomics, often abbreviated "PGx" is the study of the role of the genome in drug response. Its name reflects its combining of pharmacology and genomics. Pharmacogenomics is the study of how genes affect a person's response to drugs. This field combines pharmacology (the science of drugs) and genomics (the study of genes and their functions) to develop effective, safe medications that can be prescribed based on a person's genetic makeup. The main objectives of this work - Develop rational means to optimize drug therapy, with regard to the patient's genotype, to achieve maximum efficiency with minimal adverse effect and Improve patient's health by helping you know ahead of time whether a drug is likely to benefit you and be safe to use for the patient. Purpose of Research in Pharmacogenomics is to define these genetic mechanisms, and ultimately to implement genetic testing to improve drug efficacy and reduce toxicity, for example: The antiretroviral drug Abacavir, used in the treatment of HIV/AIDS. About 5% of people will have a severe hypersensitivity reaction of this drug, which in some cases is life threatening. Conclusion is hence the pharmacogenomics helps to develop drugs which is compatible with the patient's genome.

Keywords: *Pharmacogenomics1, genetic mechanisms2, adverse effects3, Abacavir4, hypersensitivity5*

Presented as Poster

Trigeminal Neuralgia

Scan to View online

Presented by
Pushpa Satya Mahalakshmi Sanivarapu, Priyanka Rambbudi, Divya Merugu
Aditya Pharmacy College, Aditya University, Surampalem, Andhra Pradesh, India

Abstract

A sudden, intense, transient, stabbing, and recurring pain in one or more trigeminal nerve branches is known as trigeminal neuralgia (tn).tn also known as trigeminal neuralgia, formerly called tic douloureux, is typified by recurring, short bursts of electric shock-like pain that impact the regions innervated by the fifth cranial nerve (cn). Cn v, the trigeminal nerve, innervates the lower jaw, face, and forehead. Though it can affect one or more trigeminal nerve divisions, unilateral trigeminal neuralgia is the most common type. Information about touch, pain, and temperature is transmitted from the ipsilateral face to the contralateral thalamus by the trigeminothalamic tract, which is made up of peripheral sensory components that converge at the trigeminal ganglia. There are three divisions of the trigeminal nerve: the mandibular (v3), maxillary (v2), and ophthalmic (v1). Different clinical, pathological, and prognostic entities are represented by type 1 pain, which is intermittent, and type 2 pain, which is persistent. Neurovascular conflict is the most widely recognized explanation, despite the possibility of other mechanisms involving peripheral diseases at the root (compression or traction), as well as dysfunctions of the brain stem, basal ganglion, and cortical pain modulatory mechanisms. The diagnosis is primarily made clinically; magnetic resonance imaging (mri) can be used to identify pathological alterations in the afflicted root and neurovascular compression (nvc), as well as to rule out secondary causes.

Keywords: *Trigeminal Neuralgia, Neurovascular Compression, Trigeminothalamic Tract, Tic Douloureux, Neurovascular Conflict*

Presented as Poster

Intermittent Fasting As An Adjunctive Strategy For Diabetes Management

Scan to View online

Presented by
Singampalli Pravallika
Aditya Pharmacy College, Aditya University, Surampalem, Andhra Pradesh, India

Abstract

Intermittent fasting (if) has emerged as a noteworthy approach for the management of type 2 diabetes mellitus (t2dm), a chronic disorder often marked by diminished insulin sensitivity or insufficient insulin production, resulting in impaired glucose regulation. This review explores the physiological effects of if on metabolic health, particularly its influence on blood glucose levels, insulin sensitivity, and weight management, drawing on evidence from both animal studies and human clinical trials. Additionally, some investigations indicate that if could further reduce insulin requirements, potentially benefiting patients who aim to decrease their reliance on medication. While the potential advantages of if are compelling, it is essential to acknowledge the associated risks, especially for individuals with diabetes, which necessitates a cautious approach. Current research presents varied outcomes regarding the long-term effects of if on insulin resistance and hba1c levels, underscoring the need for further investigation to fully ascertain its efficacy. Intermittent fasting may improve diabetes management by enhancing glucose regulation and metabolic health. Current studies highlight the need for personalized and closely monitored approaches to ensure safety and effectiveness, as individual responses to fasting can vary significantly.

Keywords: *Intermittent Fasting, Type 2 Diabetes Mellitus, Insulin Resistance, Glycemic Control, Weight Management, Diabetes Treatment*

Presented as Poster

Booming Of 3D Printing Technology

Scan to View online

Presented by
S. Prasanthi, Sk.Rasheedha, K.Neelima
School of Pharmaceutical Sciences & Technologies, JNTU, Kakinada, Andhra Pradesh, India

Abstract

Three - dimensional printing technology is an Additive manufacturing technology, focusing on development of personalised medicine. Spirtam (levetiracetam) was the first 3D printed prescription drug to be approved by the Food and Drug Administration (FDA) in August 2015. It enables us to produce the preparations with complex structures and preparations with precise control release of drugs. By using this technology, it is possible to develop the patient - specific medicines that meet the individual needs by enhancing patient compliance. The patient-specific medications like implants can be printed using the patient's own cells to increase biocompatibility and 3D printed organs can be developed for drug testing and study of toxicity of newer medications. This technology allows the preparations with multiple active ingredients in a single dosage form. Due to its immense applications and potential in the pharmaceutical and healthcare sector, it has earned much attention. Despite its potential, it also has challenges regarding the regulation and ensuring the safety and efficacy of drugs. The higher benefits over the disadvantages gives a broad perspective of future reliance of the pharmaceutical Applications on 3D printing technology.

Keywords: *3 D printing technology, Additive manufacturing, Personalised medicine, Spirtam, 3D Printed organs.*

Presented as Poster

Super Computer Based Approaches To Rational Drug Design

Scan to View online

Presented by
Moturi Satya Sindhu Priya
VJ's College of Pharmacy, Rajahmundry,
Andhra Pradesh, India

Abstract

We present a supercomputer-driven pipeline for in-silico drug discovery using enhanced sampling molecular dynamics (MD) and ensemble docking. Ensemble docking makes use of MD results by docking compound databases into representative protein binding-site conformations, thus taking into account the dynamic properties of the binding sites. We also describe preliminary results obtained for 23 systems involving eight proteins of the proteome of SARS-CoV-2. The MD involves temperature replica exchange enhanced sampling, making use of massively-parallel supercomputing to quickly sample the configurational space of protein drug targets. Using the Summit supercomputer at the Oak Ridge National Laboratory, more than 1 ms of enhanced sampling MD can be generated per day.

Keywords: *Molecular docking, pharmacophore modelling, virtual screening, molecular dynamics,QSAR analysis*

Presented as Poster

Green Chemistry : A Waste Management Strategy

Scan to View online

Presented by
M.Prasanna Lakshmi, R.Harshitha Valli, K.Sirisha, R.Sirisha
Sri Vasavi Institute of Pharmaceutical Sciences, Pedatadepalli, Andhra Pradesh, India

Abstract

Green chemistry refers to the creation, development, and application of chemical products and procedures that minimize or completely do away with the usage and production of compounds that are harmful to the environment and human health. The application of organic solvents in sample preparation is examined in relation to the "reduce, replace, and remove" tenets of green chemistry. Here discusses the application of GAC principles in pharmaceutical analysis, with an emphasis on direct analytical techniques that involve little to no sample preparation, "the most polluting" step, and research that either minimizes the use of hazardous solvents or substitutes them with safer, more environmentally friendly solvents.In terms of energy consumption, operator safety, and ecological impact, environmentally friendly HPLC procedures perform better than conventional methods. Additionally, they provide improved technique performance, which encourages the pharmaceutical industry to embrace the Green Analytical Chemistry (GAC) methodology. Analysts, the pharmaceutical industry, and the micro community all gain from the application of green principles in drug analysis. Starting again and developing whole new analytical techniques isn't usually required. By adopting a more environmentally conscious mindset, all current analytical techniques can be adjusted to meet the demands of green chemistry.

Keywords: *Green chemistry, Pharmaceutical industry, HPLC, Green solvents, Drug analysis*

Presented as Poster

Humanization Strategies In ICU: Balancing Technology And Compassionate Care

Scan to View online

Presented by
Hepzibah Rani Gidla, Dr. D. Sathis Kumar, Dr. Pavan Kumar Yanamadala
Aditya Pharmacy College, Aditya University, Surampalem, Andhra Pradesh, India

Abstract

Intensive care units (icus) play a crucial role in the stabilization of patients facing critical health challenges; however, the growing dependence on sophisticated medical technologies has sparked concerns regarding the potential depersonalization of care. In contemporary settings, there is often a predominant focus on clinical protocols, which can overshadow the psychological and emotional requirements of both patients and their families, resulting in a pervasive sense of dehumanization. Research has shown that individuals in icus frequently experience feelings of isolation and objectification, primarily attributed to insufficient communication, a diminished sense of personal agency, and an emphasis on their medical conditions rather than their overall human experience. Allowing unrestricted visiting hours and clear communication can help families cope during critical times. However, healthcare providers often experience moral distress and burnout due to the pressures of their roles. The goal is to transform icus into spaces that prioritize not just survival but also healing and interpersonal connections, ultimately improving patient satisfaction and creating a nurturing environment for families while balancing medical demands with compassion and dignity.

Keywords: *Intensive Care Unit (ICU), Humanization, Patient Dignity, Family Involvement, Healthcare Worker Well-being, Psychological Outcomes*

Presented as Poster

Multi-Layer Tablet

Scan to View online

Presented by
M.Tanusree, P.Triveni
Raghu College of Pharmacy,
Bheemunipatnam, Andhra Pradesh, India

Abstract

Multi-layer tablet is a new era for winning development of controlled release formulation along with various features to provide successful drug delivery. Bi-layer tablets can be crucial option to incompatibilities avoid chemical between active pharmaceutical ingredients (APIs) by physical separation and to facilitate the development of different drug release profiles. Multi-layer tablet is appropriate for chronological release of two drugs in combination and also for sustained release of tablet in which one layer is for immediate release as loading dose and second layer is maintenance dose. So use of bi-layer tablets is a very different aspect for anti-hypertensive, diabetic, anti-inflammatory and analgesic drugs where combination therapy is often used

Keywords: *Multicoated tablets, bilayer tablets,API,loading dose, maintanence dose , combination therapy*

Presented as Poster

Nanobots In Cancer: Pioneering Precision And Targeted Cancer Therapy

Scan to View online

Presented by
Sk.Saniya Meerza
Srinivasa Rao College of Pharmacy,
Visakhapatnam, Andhra Pradesh, India

Abstract

Nanobots are nano-scale machines designed to perform specific tasks at the cellular level. In cancer treatment, nanobots hold immense potential due to their ability to precisely target cancer cells, minimizing damage to surrounding healthy tissue. Nanotechnology in cancer treatment is advancing from research to clinical applications. Nanobots can be programmed to deliver drugs, detect cancerous cells, or directly destroy tumors. They can identify molecular markers on cancer cells, allowing for highly targeted interventions, and can release drugs in a controlled manner to enhance treatment efficacy. Some nanobots are equipped with materials that react to external stimuli (e.g., magnetic fields or light) to generate heat and destroy cancer cells. Diagnostic nanobots can detect cancer biomarkers in the bloodstream at very early stages, aiding in early intervention. With ongoing research, nanobots may soon be able to self-navigate and carry multiple therapeutic agents, offering combined treatment and diagnostic (theranostic) capabilities. Integrating artificial intelligence may further enhance precision and adaptability in personalized cancer treatment. Nanobot technology in oncology is revolutionizing how we approach cancer treatment, moving towards personalized, less invasive, and highly effective therapeutic strategies. Continued advancements could make nanobots a central tool in future cancer care.

Keywords: *Cancer detection, Nanobots, Theraputic methods, Drug delivery, Tumor sensing , Targeted therapy*

Presented as Poster

Transungual Drug Delivery System

Scan to View online

Presented by
T.L Bhavya Sri, Mohammad Ahmadunnisa, P.Haripriya,T.Bhagya Sri
Sri Vasavi Institute of Pharmaceutical Sciences, Pedatadepalli, Andhra Pradesh, India

Abstract

A drug delivery system is defined as a technological formulation that facilitates the administration of a drug molecule into the body while controlling the rate, extent, and location of drug release. Transungual drug delivery specifically targets the nail plate, enabling effective treatment for nail disorders. Conventional treatments, such as oral and topical medications, often come with undesirable side effects, high relapse rates, and limited efficacy. Recent advancements in nail drug delivery systems (NDDS) are transforming therapeutic approaches by integrating cutting-edge technologies that enable precise, controlled, and targeted medication delivery. These innovations address key challenges, such as inadequate drug penetration due to the nail's structure and loss of topical formulations from washing or rubbing, which can lead to uneven drug distribution. The review explores both established and emerging methods for diagnosing and treating nail infections and disorders. By investigating these approaches, this review seeks to ensure therapeutic efficacy and enhance drug penetration to deeper layers of this complex structure. Additionally, it includes a discussion of current treatments and therapies under clinical trial.

Keywords: *Transungual delivery, therapeutic, nanoparticles,bio adhesive,nail lacquer , polymeric*

Presented as Poster

A Comprehensive Review Of AI-Powered Chatbot Interventions For Chronic Illness Management

Scan to View online

Presented by
Mercy Pinipe, Dr. M. Phani Ramana Bushan
Aditya Pharmacy College, Aditya University, Surampalem, Andhra Pradesh, India

Abstract

The use of AI in chatbots for chronic diseases has become increasingly important for enhancing patient communication and addressing the growing demand for supportive healthcare. However, there is a lack of comprehensive reviews on the impact of ai-driven chatbot interventions in healthcare literature. This research aimed to evaluate user satisfaction, intervention effectiveness, and the specific features and ai frameworks of chatbots designed for chronic diseases. A thorough literature review was conducted across several databases, including pubmed and scopus, focusing on studies that used chatbots or ai frameworks for preventing, treating, or rehabilitating chronic diseases. The review also assessed bias risk using the risk of bias 2.0 tools. Out of 784 identified results, eight studies met the inclusion criteria, focusing on various intervention strategies: health education (3), behavior change theory (1), stress and coping (1), cognitive behavioral therapy (2), and self-care behavior (1). The research revealed that ai-driven chatbots are effective and user-friendly for managing chronic conditions, with users generally expressing positive acceptance of these tools for self-management. Future studies should focus on detailed descriptions and patient safety, using natural language processing and multimodal interaction. Evidence-based assessments are needed to facilitate comparisons across different chronic health conditions.

Keywords: *Artificial intelligence, chatbot, chronic illness, conversational agents.*

Presented as Poster

Concept Of Social Pharmacy

Scan to View online

Presented by
S.Sri Vyshnavi , Sk .Karishma Begum, D.Geetha,D.Amrutha Varshini
Sri Vasavi Institute of Pharmaceutical Sciences, Pedatadepalli, Andhra Pradesh, India

Abstract

Social pharmacy is a multidisciplinary field of study that examines the role of medicines in society from social, scientific, and humanistic perspectives. It includes the study of the social, economic, and organizational aspects of medicines, as well as the function, availability, control, and application of drugs in society. The interdisciplinary discipline of social pharmacy is concerned with the behavioural, social, and economic facets of drug use and pharmacy practice. Health outcomes, medication adherence, and the overall efficacy of pharmacological care are all examined in relation to socioeconomic issues. Important topics of interest consist of: Patient behaviour is the comprehension of the ways in which social influences, attitudes, and beliefs impact health behaviours and medication compliance. Examining how access to healthcare, socioeconomic status, and culture affect medicine use and health consequences is known as health disparities. Pharmacy Practice: Assessing how chemists may improve patient care and advance public health via community outreach and education. Examining healthcare policies that impact access to medications, cost, and care quality is known as policy and advocacy. Promoting cooperation between communities and chemists to solve health needs. In general, social pharmacy seeks to improve pharmacological care's efficacy by incorporating social science viewpoints into pharmacy practice.

Keywords: *patient behaviour ,pharmacological care ,socioeconomic status , multidisciplinary studies*

Presented as Poster

Revolutionizing Antibiotic Therapy: The Rise Of Zosurabalpin And Role Of Cad In Its Drug Design

Scan to View online

Presented by
K.B.Shashank
VJ's College of Pharmacy, Rajahmundry, Andhra Pradesh, India

Abstract

The everyday concern and rise in the evolution of the microorganisms leads to the heavy and intense usage of the antibiotics leads to their resistance. So there is requirement of the antibiotic resistant drugs to be designed and formulated to solve this medical issue. The drug discovery and development process aim to design compounds with optimized efficacy, safety, and pharmacokinetic properties. Zosurabalpin is a newly synthesized therapeutic agent developed for the treatment of multidrug-resistant bacterial infections. Its design is based on the structural optimization of a lead compound identified through high-throughput screening and computational modelling. Structure-activity relationship (SAR) studies were conducted to identify key functional groups and optimize the pharmacophore for enhanced efficacy. Molecular docking and dynamics simulations were employed to predict the binding affinity and stability of Zosurabalpin with its bacterial targets. The synthetic pathway was optimized for yield, purity, and scalability. Zosurabalpin demonstrated potent *in-vitro* antibacterial activity against a range of multidrug-resistant bacterial strains, including MRSA and carbapenem-resistant Enterobacteriaceae. Molecular docking studies revealed a high binding affinity of Zosurabalpin to bacterial penicillin-binding proteins (PBPs) and DNA gyrase, suggesting a dual mechanism of action.

Keywords: *Zosurabalpin,multi drug resistant, penicillin binding proteins*

Presented as Poster

A Pharmacological Evaluation For The Ethanolic Extract Of Ipomoea Sagittifolia For Its Antioxidant, Anti - Inflammatory And Analgesic Activities

Scan to View online

Presented by
Dr. N. Sai Krishna, K.V.S. Koundinya,
Ch. Sri Chakradhar, M. Srinivasu
AKRG College Of Pharmacy, Nallajerla,
Andhra Pradesh

Abstract

This study evaluates the phytochemical, antioxidant, anti-inflammatory, and analgesic properties of the ethanolic extract from the leaves of Ipomoea sagittifolia. Phytochemical screening revealed the presence of carbohydrates, proteins, cardiac glycosides, flavonoids, tannins, and phenols. The antioxidant activity was confirmed through a hydrogen peroxide scavenging assay, achieving 92.61% inhibition at 400 μg/ml. The extract also demonstrated potent anti-inflammatory effects, inhibiting 78.26% protein denaturation, and providing 80.08% membrane stabilization in rabbit red blood cells. In *in vivo* studies, the carrageenan-induced paw edema model showed 46.4% inhibition of paw swelling after five hours at a dose of 400 mg/kg. Additionally, the analgesic potential was validated through Eddy's hot plate test, showing increased paw withdrawal latency in mice. These results suggest that the ethanolic extract of Ipomoea sagittifolia could serve as a therapeutic agent for treating conditions associated with oxidative stress, inflammation, and pain. Further research is required to isolate the active compounds and explore their mechanisms of action.

Keywords: *Ipomoea sagittifolia, ethanolic extract, antioxidant activity, anti-inflammatory, analgesic activity, oxidative stress, carrageenan-induced paw edema, herbal medicine.*

Presented as Poster

Artificial Intelligence In Preclinical Studies

Scan to View online

Presented by
Y.Lokesh, P.Rama Harini
Krishna University – College of Pharmaceutical Sciences and Research, Rudravaram, Andhra Pradesh, India

Abstract

Artificial intelligence (AI) is becoming an integral part of drug discovery. It has the potential to deliver across the drug discovery and development value chain, starting from target identification and reaching through clinical development. In this review, we provide an overview of current AI technologies and a glimpse of how AI is reimagining preclinical drug discovery by highlighting examples where AI has made a real impact. we aim to present a realistic view by discussing both opportunities and challenges in adopting AI in drug discovery. Machine Learning (ML) is a specific subset of AI that addresses this ability and enables machines and their software to learn from experience.

Keywords: *Artificial Intelligence, Drug discovery, Machine learning*

Presented as Poster

Digital Therapeutics

Scan to View online

Presented by
T.Mani Swetha, V Renuka Sri Priya
VJ's College of Pharmacy, Rajahmundry, Andhra Pradesh, India

Abstract

Digital therapeutics (DTX) represent a burgeoning field at the intersection of healthcare and technology, offering innovative solutions for managing and treating various medical conditions. These software- based interventions leverage the power of digital tools, such as mobile apps and wearables, to deliver evidence-based therapies and interventions. This abstract provides an overview of the key concepts, potential benefits, and challenges associated with digital therapeutics. It explores their role in revolutionizing healthcare delivery, improving patient outcomes, and reshaping the traditional pharmaceutical landscape. Additionally, it discusses regulatory considerations and future prospects for this rapidly evolving field.

Keywords: *Mobile health, digital therapeutics, pharmacy practice*

Presented as Poster

Advances In Parkinson'S Disease Management: Continuous Subcutaneous Foslevodopa - Foscarbidopa

Scan to View online

Presented by
G.Uha Naga Pallavi
Srinivasa Rao College of Pharmacy,
Visakhapatnam, Andhra Pradesh, India

Abstract

Parkinson's disease (PD) is a progressive neurological disorder marked by motor and non-motor symptoms, mainly due to the loss of dopamine-producing neurons. Long-term use of levodopa, the standard treatment, often leads to fluctuating effects and dyskinesia, highlighting the need for alternative therapies. A systematic search was conducted up to November 2023 in databases like PubMed, Web of Science, and Cochrane Library, yielding eight relevant studies, including pharmacological research, case reports, observational studies, and controlled trials, without language limitations. Foslevodopa and foscarbidopa, as prodrugs of levodopa and carbidopa, have excellent stability and solubility, enabling continuous subcutaneous infusion. Clinical trials show that these prodrugs maintain stable levodopa levels, effectively addressing the limitations of oral levodopa therapy. Foslevodopa-foscarbidopa shows promise as an alternative treatment for advanced PD, offering consistent symptom control and effective management of motor fluctuations and dyskinesia. Further research should explore long-term safety, cost-effectiveness, and wider accessibility. Foslevodopa-foscarbidopa is now commercially available in several European countries and Japan.

Keywords: *Parkinson's disease, Foslevodopa -foscarbidopa, continuous subcutaneous infusion,motor fluctuations,dyskinesias,levodopa therapy*

Presented as Poster

Formulation Of Controlled-Release Tablets Of Dapagliflozin Using Locust Bean Gum As A Natural Retardant

Scan to View online

Presented by

Udaya Kumar Thummala, Chitneedi Lakshmi Geethika, Hitesh Raj Mandal
Aditya Pharmacy College, Aditya University, Surampalem, Andhra Pradesh, India

Abstract

The purpose of this research was to formulate controlled-release dapagliflozin tablets using locust bean gum as a natural release retardant. Locust bean gum was purified and incorporated into tablet formulations at concentrations of 5%, 10%, and 15% using direct compression. Drug release was evaluated over 24 hours. Results showed that the 15% locust bean gum formulation effectively prolonged drug release, demonstrating sustained release over the study period. This work suggests that locust bean gum can serve as an effective natural release retardant in controlled-release tablet formulations, providing a green alternative to synthetic excipients.

Keywords: *Dapagliflozin, Locust Bean Gum, Controlled-Release, Natural Retardant, Tablet Formu*

Presented as Poster

Omics Data Integration

Scan to View online

Presented by
Bhavyasri Nandipati
Aditya Pharmacy College, Aditya University, Surampalem, Andhra Pradesh, India

Abstract

The method of multi-omics integration from various biomolecular levels, including proteins, metabolites, dna, rna, and epigenetic markers, presents detailed information of how biological systems work and respond. Multi-omics has been used in the case of various tasks such as the discovery of novel medications, the identification of new diseases, changing the therapy, and optimisation of existing ones. Invention of new biomarkers and therapeutic targets for various diseases, including cancers, can be achieved by multi-omics integration, which includes information from multiple omics levels, including the genome, transcriptome, proteome, metabolome, and microbiome. Combination of many omics results in the showing of relationships and interactions between molecular entities and biological processes. Due to variations in protein shapes and functions that can be impacted by gene expression, alternative splicing, post-translational modifications, protein-protein interactions, and protein degradation, proteome complexity can be a challenge to the design of therapeutic interventions. However, the act of combining data for multi-omics research is critical and time-consuming, requiring very well preparation and execution of study design, data creation, data processing, data analysis, and data interpretation. The invention and usage of certain techniques and apparatus that can surely and perfectly integrate multi-omics data are also necessary.

Keywords: *Multi-omics, Cancers, Multi-omics integration, Proteome complexity, Molecular entities.*

Presented as Poster

Statistical Optimisation Of Natural Gums In Development Of Extended Release Matrix Tablets Using D Optimal Mixture Design

Scan to View online

Presented by
Mr. P.N.Mallikarjun
Vignan Institute of Pharmaceutical Technology, Visakhapatnam, Andhra Pradesh, India

Abstract

The objective of this current research was to create and fine tune extended-release glipizide tablets, with a focus on utilizing natural gums, Lannea coromandelica gum (LCG) and Terminalia catappa gum (TCG), as agents to control drug release using D optimal mixture design.Glipizide is widely used anti diabetic and BCS II drug The tablet formulation was prepared by wet granulation method and the formulation optimization was done by D-optimal mixture design using Design Expert® software. The independent variables studied were LCG (X1), TCG (X2) and lactose monohydrate (X3) taking various combinations gums.The dependent (responses) variables studied were T50% (R1), T90% (R2), Drug release at 2 hrs (R3) and MDT (R4). For optimization studies, the response surface plots were generated and the optimized formulation was selected on the basis of maximum desirability value. All the evaluated parameters of all the formulations were within the pharmacopoeial limits.All formulated tablets drug release fitted into various kinetic models and most of formulations followed first order. The optimized tablet formulation was found to possess all physical properties within the desired range and showed extended release profile with 99% drug release in 24 h duration. The findings suggested that natural gums-based matrix tablets of glipizide could be successfully developed and natural gums can be explored as platform technology as release retardants and in the development of extended-release matrix tablets of other drugs.

Keywords: *D optimal,Lannea coramondelica,Terminalia catappa,MDT,T50%,T90%*

Presented as Oral Presentation

Antimicrobial Stewardship In Action: Reducing Resistance And Hospital Infections In A Tertiary Care Facility

Scan to View online

Presented by
Dr. Nandini Palivela
Aditya College of Pharmacy, Aditya University, Surampalem, Andhra Pradesh, India

Abstract

This study aimed to evaluate the effectiveness of a comprehensive antimicrobial stewardship (AS) intervention in a 500-bed tertiary care hospital to address the global challenge of antimicrobial resistance (AMR). Over six months, the intervention included multidisciplinary rounds led by infectious disease specialists, establishing antimicrobial prescribing guidelines and educational sessions for healthcare providers. A total of 1,200 patients, split evenly into pre- and post-intervention groups, were analyzed. The findings revealed a 30% decrease in antimicrobial consumption, significant reductions in broad-spectrum antibiotic use ($p < 0.01$), a 25% drop in Clostridium difficile infections, and a 15% reduction in hospital-acquired infections ($p < 0.05$). Resistance rates for pathogens like Escherichia coli and Staphylococcus aureus also declined. These results underscore the value of comprehensive AS programs in optimizing antimicrobial use, improving patient outcomes, and combatting AMR. The study provides important insights for healthcare institutions, while further research is needed to explore the long-term impact of such interventions on AMR trends.

Keywords: *Antimicrobial Resistance, Antimicrobial stewardship, Hospital-acquired infections, Tertiary care hospital, patient outcomes*

Presented as Oral Presentation

Synthesis, Anti Bacterial Activity And Molecular Docking Studies Of Some New 4-Tert-Butyl Chalcones Against Multidrug Resistant Pathogens

Scan to View online

Presented by
Mr. A.Kanaka Raju
Vignan Institute of Pharmaceutical Technology, Visakhapatnam, Andhra Pradesh, India

Abstract

The rising threat of drug-resistant microbes highlights the critical need for new antimicrobial agents. To tackle this issue, significant research efforts have focused on developing innovative strategies and frameworks. Chalcones, recognized for their broad-spectrum biological activities, have emerged as promising candidates in the fight against drug resistance. In this study synthesized a series of 4-tert-butyl chalcones (R1 to R15) with varying electron-withdrawing and electron-donating groups using Claisen-Schmidt condensation. The structures of the synthesized compounds were confirmed through FT-IR, 1H NMR, and 13C NMR analysis. Evaluation of these compounds revealed their potential as antibacterial agents, with compounds R2 and R9 demonstrating strong antibacterial activity against multidrug-resistant (MDR) bacteria, including E. coli, P. aeruginosa, K. pneumoniae, and S. aureus, outperforming the reference drug Ciprofloxacin. Additionally, molecular docking studies using Auto Dock Vina molecular docking software for Glucosamine-6-phosphate (GlcN-6-P) synthase inhibition indicated that ligands R2 and R9 exhibited impressive binding energy values of −12 kcal/mol and −11 kcal/mol respectively, correlating with their antibacterial activity. These results highlight the potential of chalcones, particularly R2 and R9, as promising candidates for developing new antimicrobial agents targeting drug-resistant microbes.

Keywords: *chalcones, antibacterial activity, molecular docking, (GlcN-6-P) synthase inhibition*

Presented as Oral Presentation

Advances In Crispr-Based Organoid Models For Studying Hereditary Kidney Diseases.

Scan to View online

Presented by
Miss Bommeti Sara Aiswarya
Aditya Pharmacy College, Aditya University, Surampalem, Andhra Pradesh, India

Abstract

Gene technology, CRISPR-Cas9(Clustered Regularly Interspaced Short Palindromic Repeats- CRISPR-associated protein 9), is always challenging as it represents a revolutionary approach toward the treatment of hereditary kidney diseases, autosomal dominant polycystic kidney disease, and Alport syndrome. This technology can change the DNA sequence of the genetic mutation; therefore, it significantly advances curative treatments in a patient suffering from hereditary kidney disease. These experimental techniques on animal models of these diseases performed well in suppressing cyst formation, fibrosis, and proteinuria of the kidneys. However, difficulties remain regarding the specific delivery of the CRISPR components to the kidney tissue. Nanoparticles and viral vectors are some of the more complex delivery systems studied with tighter targeting specificity and a reduced off-target effect. Several issues regarding efficiency, safety, and specific ethical implications will have to be solved before CRISPR can be put in place on a wide scale at the level of ethical and safety issues as well as long-term clinical implications. More studies will be needed before the technical as well as ethical challenges are resolved to allow CRISPR to find its place in nephrology on a wide scale. However, the CRISPR potential is transformative and may soon be realized shortly when personalized curative therapies for genetic kidney disorders start to increasingly feature in medical treatments.

Keywords: *CRISPR-Cas9, Alport syndrome, Nanoparticles, polycystic kidney disease, Hereditary kidney disease, Fibrosis.*

Presented as Oral Presentation

Effect Of Bacopa Monnieri On Fibrinolytic Activity By Invitro Method

Scan to View online

Presented by
Mrs. Singineddi Sruthi
Aditya College of Pharmacy, Aditya University, Surampalem, Andhra Pradesh, India

Abstract

Fibrinolysis is a normal body process .fibrinolysis is the breakdown of blood clots .which is a crucial part of wound healing .if fibrinolysis is a not properly regulated can lead to numberous different diseases .collection of plant leaves of bacopa monnieri. The fibrinolytic system and its measurements ,bacopa monnieri a nootropic drug ,fibrinolysis and the control of blood coagulation . these drugs are tissue plasminogen activators ,streptokinase ,alteplase ,reteplase ,tenecteplase ,urokinase ,pro-urokinase . Preliminary phytochemical tests ,test for alkaloids ,test for tannins ,test for glycosides ,test for amino acids ,test for saponins. Formation of clots ,collect the 6ml of blood were withdrawn from the healthy volunteers and irrespective of gender . the blood was distributed into 6 previously weighed micro centrifuge tubes 1ml in each centrifuge tube .the centrifuge tubes were incubated in stimulated body temperature at 37 c for 45 minutes in heat controlled incubator .the formation of blood clots were observed. *In-vitro* fibrinolytic activity results, by the addition of 3 groups ,group 1 , group 2 , group 3 , we observed the following results , visual inspection -there is blood dissolution in group -1 and group -3 was observed. From the experimental methods we conclude that the test drug of bacopa monnieri shows the thrombolytic activity due to the presence of active ingredients like saponins alkaloids , carbohydrates ,amino acids and it a was tested for fibrinolysis by vitro methods.

Keywords: *fibrinolysis ,bacopa monnieri ,streptokinase ,fibrinolytic activity ,in-vitro method*

Presented as Oral Presentation

A Review On Liquid Crystals In Pharmacy

Scan to View online

Presented by
Mrs. Sesha Sai Durga Manyam
Aditya College of Pharmacy, Aditya University, Surampalem, Andhra Pradesh, India

Abstract

Although liquid crystalline materials are sometimes thought of as an odd state of matter, they have had a significant impact on contemporary technology. Liquid crystals, which have their origins in cholesterol derivatives, are a material that biomedical engineers and biologists deal with regularly. Since liquid crystal systems have distinct microstructures and physicochemical characteristics, they are garnering a lot of interest. Researchers and developers working in the formulation development field are increasingly choosing liquid crystals as their system of choice. A liquid crystal system can be used to efficiently deliver drugs to desired biological targets. Three factors contribute to the formation of liquid crystalline phases: chirality, microsegregation effects, and molecular shape. The purpose of this review was to give an overview of the many types of liquid crystal systems and how they are prepared. Pharmaceutical liquid crystals and their significance in targeted drug delivery systems are to be scientifically highlighted in this review paper. This review's primary goal is to give comprehensive information on pharmaceutical liquid crystal technology, including the most recent and cutting-edge technological advancements.

Keywords: *liquid crystals,lyotorpic crystal, thermo tropic crystal,*

Presented as Oral Presentation

Preparation And Characterization Of Mouth Dissolving Tablets Of Indomethacin Using Banana Peel Powder As A Natural Super Disintegrant

Scan to View online

Presented by
Miss Ketha Srilekhya
Vignan Institute of Pharmaceutical Technology, Visakhapatnam, Andhra Pradesh, India

Abstract

Mouth dissolving tablets are meant for administration to the patients who cannot swallow, such as elderly, stroke victims, bedridden patients, patients affected by renal failure, and the patients who refuse to swallow, such as pediatric, geriatric, and psychiatric patients. The aim of the study is to formulate mouth dissolving tablet of Indomethacin for the pain management of Rheumatoid Arthritis and to improve the efficacy and patient compliance. In the present work, fast dissolving tablets of Indomethacin were prepared by direct compression method using Banana peel powder as natural super disintegrant with a view to enhance patient compliance and to avoid hepatic first pass metabolism and to improve its bioavailability. The prepared formulations of tablets were evaluated for hardness,thickness, friability, drug content uniformity, wetting time, disintegration and *In vivo* dissoution studies.Thus the study leads that Musa paradisicum (Banana peel powder)releases high amount of drug content which is used as natural super disintegrant.

Keywords: *Mouth dissolving tablets, Indomethacin, Musa Paradisicum, Rheumatoid Arthritis, Natural super disintegrant*

Presented as Oral Presentation

Estimation Of Anti-Hyperglycaemic Effect Of Glochidion Tomentosum In Stz Induced Diabetic Rats

Scan to View online

Presented by
Dr. K Daniel Raju
Vignan Institute of Pharmaceutical Technology, Visakhapatnam, Andhra Pradesh, India

Abstract

Glochidion tomentosum has traditionally been used as antimicrobial, anthelmintic, antioxidant and research is going on various other properties of the plant including diabetes mellitus. The plant extract consists of majorly terpenoids, tannins, alkaloids, glycosides, and steroids. The purpose of this study was to investigate the antidiabetic activity of the plant Glochidion tomentosum streptozotocin (STZ) induced diabetic rats. The administration of STZ (55mg/kg) significantly ($p<0.001$) increased the Fasting blood sugar level when compared to the normal control group. The fasting blood sugar level, food intake & water intake are increased in diabetes control group, whereas the body weight is decreased in diabetes control group after the STZ administration. After successive treatment with Glochidion tomentosum 21 days, the over said increased parameters are decreased significantly ($p<0.01$) and the body weight is maintained to normal control group. The overall results indicated that Glochidion tomentosum has almost equivalent antidiabetic potential and might be due to its insulinotropic action which increases the utilization of glucose thoroughly inside the body. The presence of glycosides, tannins, alkaloids, steroids, terpenoids in selected plant might be responsible for its therapeutic effect.

Keywords: *Glochidion tomentosum, Insulinotropic, Antidiabetic, Streptozotocin, Type-2 Diabetes*

Presented as Oral Presentation

Comparative Assay Screening Of Lapatinib By Uv Spectroscopy And Liquid Chromatography

Scan to View online

Presented by
Dr. Bhagavan Rajesh Babu Koppisetty
Vignan Institute of Pharmaceutical Technology, Visakhapatnam, Andhra Pradesh, India

Abstract

A simple, rapid and sensitive validated UV-Spectrophotometry and RP-liquid chromatographic method have been developed for the assay of Lapatinib in Bulk and Pharmaceutical dosage form. Chromatographic separation achieved on a C18 SpolarG 250×4.6mm column in Isocratic elution with mobile phase containing water methanol, acetonitrile in ratio(75 : 15 : 10 v/v). The flow rate was 1 mL/min and effluent were monitored at 235nm. The elution/retention time of Lapatinib at 6.01 min. LOD and LOQ forHPLC method was 0.125 μg/mL and 0.380 μg/mL respectively.U.V absorption spectra were screened in the range in between 200-400 nm and the assay for Lapatinib absorption set at λ maximum 235nm, the developed method was validated according to ICH guidelines. The linearity data of Lapatinib are 2 to 12 μg/mL, LOD and LOQ are 0.230μg/mL and 0.699μg/mL respectively. The comparative assay studies were performed using UV and liquid chromatography. The developed method was successfully applied to bulk drugs as well as in Pharmaceutical dosage form.

Keywords: *Lapatinib, UV Spectroscopy, RP-HPLC*

Presented as Oral Presentation

Spindle Cell Sarcoma (Abstract)

Scan to View online

Presented by
Dr. Penugonda Vineela
Aditya College of Pharmacy, Aditya University, Surampalem, Andhra Pradesh, India

Abstract

Spindle cell sarcoma is a very rare, malignant cancer that affects the bone or soft tissue. It is a type of connective tissue cancer that usually starts with a small and inflamed lump that grows in size. The cancer cells looks like spindles.spindle cells divide uncontrollably, forming a mass of cells that creates a tumor. The cells look long and narrow with tapered ends when viewed under a microscope. Spindle cell sarcoma can occur anywhere in the body, but most commonly occurs in the arms and legs. Causes of this cancer may not known but some risk factors that aggravate this disease includes genetic predisposition – gene irregularities have passed from parents, radiation exposure and other disease conditions like Paget's Disease of the Bone etc. symptoms include bone pain ,Pathological bone fracture due to weakening of the bone, Swelling, Tenderness or soreness, Reduced mobility in the affected area, or in a nearby joint. cancerous traits can be detected through cell-level molecular analysis. As such, at Stage 1, the tumor is usually treated by excision, includes wide margins of healthy-looking tissue, followed by thorough biopsy, and additional excision. The prognosis for a stage 1 tumor excision is usually fairly optimistic, but if the tumor progresses to levels 2 and 3, prognosis worsens, due to tumor cells' likely having spread to other parts of the body includes lungs, kidneys, and liver. In these cases, prognosis is grim and chemotherapy and radiation are the only methods of controlling the cancer.

Keywords: *Sarcoma, Spindle Cells, connective Tissue, genetic predisposition, chemotherphy*

Presented as Oral Presentation

Quercetin – A Flavonoid For Targeting Cancer

Scan to View online

Presented by
Dr. B.N.B.Vaidehi
Aditya College of Pharmacy, Aditya University, Surampalem, Andhra Pradesh, India

Abstract

Quercetin has a flavone nucleus of two benzene rings connected by a heterocyclic pyrone ring. Because animals cannot generate the nucleus of flavones, flavonoids are only found in plants. Among the many foods and plants that contain quercetin are fruits, seeds, vegetables, tea, coffee, bracken fern, and natural colors. It is Insoluble in water, mildly soluble in alcohol, and in glacial acetic acid and aqueous alkaline solutions. Quercetin is a yellow, crystalline solid with a bitter flavor. Quercetin and almost 2,000 other flavonoids are produced when p-glycosides condense. Rutin (quercetin-3-rutinoside), a naturally occurring flavonoid, is often hydrolyzed to yield quercetin. On the other hand, quercetin has a strong toxic effect on cancer cells while causing little to no harm to healthy cells. Numerous studies have demonstrated quercetin's capacity to prevent several cancers, including those of the breast, lung, nasopharynx, kidney, colon, prostate, pancreas, and ovaries. Numerous *in-vitro* and *in vivo* investigations were carried out to assess quercetin's cytotoxic effects on ovarian cancer.

Keywords: *favanoid, quercetin, hetrocyclic, rutin,cancer*

Presented as Oral Presentation

Formulation And Evaluation Of Burn Healing Ash Cream From Leaves Of *Mangifera Indica L.*

Scan to View online

Presented by
Mrs. Sadhe Amala, Leticia
Aditya College of Pharmacy, Aditya University, Surampalem, Andhra Pradesh, India

Abstract

Abstract: The present study discusses the challenges, advances and novel strategies in burn management and research with a focus on testing new pharmacological interventions in finding new targets. Besides wound healing the importance of secondary burn healing has also gained attention in the present days. The fresh leaves of Mangifera indica L were collected, dried and pulverized. The powder of leaves are taken and converted into ash by using muffle furnace at an optimum temperature. Preliminary phytochemical screening were performed using UV, FTIR and chemical tests to know the presence of secondary metabolites for ash powder. The obtained ash powder is formulated using a cream base and different evaluation parameters are performed on cream like spreadability, skin sensitivity, viscosity and pH. *In-vitro* burn healing activity was performed using albino mice for 21 days by using a standard Aminacrine and Cetrimide. The size of wound (burn) was measured as per standard protocol which indicated the test showed significance results with the standard drug. This research emphasizes the usage of herbal ash cream has the potential in burn healing might be due to the presence of antioxidant properties and anthocyanin.

Keywords: *Mangifera indica L, Ash, FTIR, Aminacrine & Cetrimide*

Presented as Oral Presentation

Targeting The Gut Microbiome: A Novel Approach To Personalized Pharmacotherapy

Scan to View online

Presented by
Miss Sarvasiddi Kiranmai
Vignan Institute of Pharmaceutical Technology, Visakhapatnam, Andhra Pradesh, India

Abstract

The gut microbiome, a complex ecosystem of microorganisms residing in the human gastrointestinal tract, has emerged as a critical player in modulating drug metabolism, efficacy, and toxicity. This presentation explores the burgeoning field of pharmacomicrobiomics, which seeks to understand the interactions between microbial communities and pharmaceutical agents. Recent studies indicate that variations in microbiome composition can lead to significant inter-individual differences in drug response, offering a potential explanation for the variable outcomes observed in treatments such as cancer therapies, cardiovascular drugs, and antibiotics. By targeting and modulating the gut microbiome, researchers are unlocking new possibilities for personalized pharmacotherapy, where drug regimens are tailored to an individual's unique microbial profile. This approach holds promise for enhancing therapeutic efficacy, reducing adverse drug reactions, and optimizing dosing strategies. As we delve deeper into the gut microbiome's role in pharmacology, it is clear that pharmacomicrobiomics will play a pivotal role in the future of personalized medicine, offering a novel frontier for improving patient outcomes and drug development strategies.

Keywords: *Gut microbiome, Pharmacomicrobiomics, Personalized pharmacotherapy, Drug metabolism, Drug efficacy.*

Presented as Oral Presentation

Formulation And *In-vitro* Evaluation Of Mouth Dissolving Tablets Of Daclatasvir Dihydrochloride

Scan to View online

Presented by
Mrs. Prasanthi Teella
Aditya College of Pharmacy, Aditya University, Surampalem, Andhra Pradesh, India

Abstract

The present study was carried out on Daclatasvir Dihydrochloride Mouth dissolving tablets were prepared by direct compression method and different concentration super disintegrants like Polyplasdone XL, Solutab and Explotab were used in mouth dissolving tablets. A total of 9 formulations were prepared and evaluated for various pre and post compression parameters like angle of repose, bulk density, tapped density, carr's index, hausner's ratio, weight variation, hardness, friability, thickness, wetting time, water absorption ratio, drug content, *in-vitro* disintegration time and *in-vitro* drug release. The *in-vitro* disintegration time of the optimised formulation (F3) of Daclatasvir Dihydrochloride was found to be 19 sec. Release rate of drug was 99.42 % within 30 minutes. FTIR studies showed good compatibility between drug and excipients.

Keywords: *Daclatasvir Dihydrochloride, Polyplasdone XL, Solutab and Explotab, Mouth dissolving tablets.*

Presented as Oral Presentation

Formulation And Characterisation Of Niosomes Encapsulating Green Tea Extract And Rosehip Oil For Enhanced Skin Care Delivery"

Scan to View online

Presented by
Mrs. A Sree Geetha
Aditya College of Pharmacy, Aditya University, Surampalem, Andhra Pradesh, India

Abstract

Niosomes, are non-ionic surfactant-based vesicular carriers, offer a promising drug delivery system to improve the bioavailability, stability, and controlled release of active ingredients. The aim of the present study is to develop a niosomal formulation that enhances the delivery of these compounds for improved skin care efficacy. Niosomes were prepared using the thin-film hydration method, employing non-ionic surfactants like Span 60 and cholesterol. Green tea extract, rich in polyphenols such as epigallocatechin gallate (EGCG), and rosehip oil, known for its vitamin C and essential fatty acid content, were incorporated into the vesicles. The formulated niosomes were characterized for their particle size, entrapment efficiency, zeta potential, and morphology using dynamic light scattering (DLS), transmission electron microscopy (TEM), and encapsulation studies. The niosomal formulation showed a particle size range of 100-200 nm with high entrapment efficiency (>85%) for both green tea extract and rosehip oil. The release studies demonstrated a sustained release profile, with more than 70% of the active compounds being released over 24 hours. The skin permeation test confirmed enhanced delivery of both the compounds. Hence the niosomal formulation containing green tea extract and rosehip oil showed promising results in terms of stability, encapsulation efficiency, and controlled release, making it a potential candidate for anti-aging and antioxidant-rich skincare products.

Keywords: *Niosomes,Anti-aging,Anti-oxidant,Green tea extract,Rose hip oil,Span 60,Skin permeation test etc*

Presented as Oral Presentation

Phytochemical Screening And Evaluation Of Antioxidant And Antipsychotic Activities Of Ethanolic Leaf Extracts Of Artemisia Pallens

Scan to View online

Presented by
Miss B.Niharika
Aditya College of Pharmacy, Aditya University, Surampalem, Andhra Pradesh, India

Abstract

Psycosis (schizophrenic, schizoaffective, and affective illness) is a group of serious illnesses that effect the mind. It is a major delibilating, complex and costly illness that strikes 1% of the world's population. It may include hallucinations, such as hearing voices (the most commonly associated symptom) or seeing things that are'nt there. Types of psychotic disorders include; Schizophrenia, Schizoaffective disorder, Bipolar disorder, Psychotic depression and Drug- induced psychosis. Here we are using an aromatic herb named (*Artemisia pallens*)which is xerophytic in nature The leaves and flowers yield an essential oil known as oil of Davana.Artemisia pallens is found abundantly in humid habitats in the plains all over india and mainly found in Nilgiri hills and has been used by the tribal people for various ailments. Oral administration of high doses aqueous extract from the aerial parts of the plants was observed to reduce blood glucose levels in glucose -fed hyperglycemic and alloxan -treated rabbits and rats. Ethanolic root extract of stem bark has been reported to possess anti-inflammatory ,analgesic activities. Ethanolic stem extract of plant is reported to possess anti-tumor and anti-bacterial activity. Oil extracted from the stem exhibits signifiicant anticancer, anti - inflammatory and anti-obesity effects.

Keywords: *Artemisiapallens, hyperlocomotion activity, tail suspension test,DPPH scavenging method, antioxidant and anti psychotic activity, davana oil .*

Presented as Oral Presentation

Formulation Optimization And Evaluation Of Herbal Films Containing Ethanol Leaves Extract Of Cassia Auriculata To Treat Chronic Constipation Disorder

Scan to View online

Presented by
Dr. A. Seetha Devi
Gokaraju Rangaraju College of Pharmacy,
Hyderabad, Telangana, India

Abstract

An intriguing trend in recent years has been the designing of oral films containing extracts from medicinal plants. Therefore, efforts were made in the current work to create fast-dissolving herbal films using Cassia auriculata ethanol leaf extract in order to create a dosage form that would be more convenient to administer and treat chronic constipation disorders in the elderly. A number of quality control measures, including weight fluctuation, thickness variation, surface pH, percentage moisture uptake, percentage moisture loss, disintegration time and folding endurance, were assessed. *In vivo* dissolving studies using Paddle type apparatus in pH 6.8 phosphate buffer pH 6.8, which is simulated saliva, were performed for each film composition. Out of all nine formulations, formulation F5, which is an herbal film with 10% propylene glycol and 40% HPMC, exhibited complete drug release (99.6%) in 30 minutes and had a strong folding endurance value. The release of medication from films was found to follow first-order kinetics. Overall, studies indicate that the most feasible dose form that can be used in medical settings for the treatment of chronic constipation disorder is fast-dissolving herbal films containing C. auriculata leaves extract. This is especially true for patients who have difficulty swallowing.

Keywords: *Herbal films, Cassia auriculata, Constipation, HPMC, Propylene glycol, Solvent casting method*

Presented as Oral Presentation

Acute Chest Syndrome In Sickle Cell Disease: A Case Report And Review Of Management Strategies

Scan to View online

Presented by
Mr. Londa Eswar Naga Sai Datta Yadav
Aditya College of Pharmacy, Aditya University, Surampalem, Andhra Pradesh, India

Abstract

Sickle cell disease (SCD) is a hereditary hematologic disorder characterized by abnormal hemoglobin leading to vaso-occlusive crises and chronic complications. This case report highlights a rare presentation of SCD in a young adult. A 25-year-old male with a known history of SCD presented to the emergency department with severe chest pain, dyspnea, and hypoxia. Chest X-ray and CT scan revealed pulmonary infarcts. Laboratory tests confirmed elevated lactate dehydrogenase (LDH) and bilirubin levels, indicating hemolysis. The patient was treated with intravenous fluids, analgesics, and blood transfusion. Despite initial improvement, he developed acute chest syndrome, requiring intensive care management and exchange transfusion. This case underscores the importance of recognizing acute chest syndrome as a potentially life-threatening complication of SCD. Timely intervention can significantly reduce morbidity and mortality. Education on early recognition and management of crises is vital for improving patient outcomes. Clinicians should maintain a high index of suspicion for acute chest syndrome in patients with SCD presenting with respiratory symptoms. Further research is needed to optimize management strategies for this condition.

Keywords: *Sickle cell disease, Acute chest syndrome, Vaso-occlusive crises, Pulmonary infarcts, Hemolysis, Blood transfusion, Patient management, Respiratory symptoms, Morbidity, Mortality*

Presented as Oral Presentation

Jogger's Nephritis Post-Pilgrimage: A Case Of Hematuria In A Devoted Pilgrim

Scan to View online

Presented by
Miss Manjari Tekumudi
Aditya Pharmacy College, Aditya University, Surampalem, Andhra Pradesh, India

Abstract

Jogger's Nephritis, or exercise-induced hematuria is an innocent condition documented in athletes with chronic exercise, including marathon running and long-distance walking. The first investigation into exercise-associated hematuria was done in the 18th century and has been attributed to several mechanisms, including renal ischemia and trauma to RBCs. Asymptomatic, nondiabetic, normotensive female patient aged 44 years who has been passing red-colored urine for 3 days. She had recently returned from a journey of 649 km to Tirumala where she covered 18.7 km General examination showed normal vitals but presented with tenderness of lower limbs on urinalysis trace albumin and 8–10 RBCs/hpf along with isomorphic RBCs. Other studies such as serum creatinine, potassium, bilirubin, and imaging were within the normal limits. Hematuria resolved spontaneously in 96 hours after rest and no RBCs were found in urine on follow-up. Management of hematuria (if painful) can be managed with mild analgesics like acetaminophen, but NSAIDs should be avoided because of renal function problems. The patient's hematuria is likely via a mechanism of renal vasoconstriction, foot strike hemolysis, and trauma to the bladder by the repeated impact of long-distance walking. This is a description of Jogger's Nephritis after strenuous exercise. It is a benign self-limiting condition, and awareness of its benign nature can also help avoid too many unnecessary interventions as much to reassure patients about the favorable prognosis.

Keywords: *Jogger's Nephritis, Hematuria, Renal Ischemia, Normotensive, Isomorphic RBCs.*

Presented as Oral Presentation

Paraganglioma

Scan to View online

Presented by
Dr. Penugonda Vineela
Aditya College of Pharmacy, Aditya University, Surampalem, Andhra Pradesh, India

Abstract

Paraganglioma is a rare neuroendocrine tumor that forms outside of the adrenal glands, which are located on top of the kidneys, they form near blood vessels and nerves, and also can be found in the neck, chest, abdomen, or pelvis. mutations in approximately 20 different genes that they think may lead to and paraganglioma. Mutations in the genes RET, VHL, NF1, SDHA, SDHB, SDHC, SDHD, CSDE1etc may play a role in forming pheochromocytoma and paragangliomas Symptoms we can see high blood pressure, fast heartbeat, sweating, headache, shaking, dizziness, flushing of the skin, nausea, pain in the back or belly, and pale appearance. Some people with this tumor have symptoms, but others don't. Symptoms may occur as often as several times in a day to a couple of times per month. Some people may feel intense symptoms that last for a short period of time called "paroxysmal attacks". These symptoms can include: High blood pressure, Headaches,Irregular heartbeat, Sweating lab tests of urine and blood to check hormone levels. imaging scans such as CT, MRI, and PET scan will done,Treatment options include medications, surgery, and radiation therapy. The definitive treatment is surgical excision of the tumor. Prognosis includes The five-year survival rate is about 95% for small paragangliomas that have not spread to other parts of the body. Some Complications my occur If left or untreated, paragangliomas can cause serious, life-threatening complications such as heart muscle disease, bleeding in the brain, accumulation of fluid in the lungs, heart attack, stroke, or coma.

Keywords: *Paraganglioma, Adrenal gland, Mutations*

Presented as Oral Presentation

Comparative Study Of Different Superdisintegrants In Designing Of Diclofenac Sodium Fast Disintegrating Tablets

Scan to View online

Presented by
Mrs. Kamma Keerthi
Aditya College of Pharmacy, Aditya University, Surampalem, Andhra Pradesh, India

Abstract

The present research work was aimed to formulate Diclofenac sodium fast disintegrating tablets using different concentrations of super disintegrants and evaluate to compare prepared formulations. Diclofenac sodium, a non steroidal anti inflammatory drug with analgesic and anti inflammatory properties was selected as a model drug. Total 9 formulations were prepared using 3 different superdisintegrants such as Sodium starch glycolate, Guar gum and croscarmellose sodium by direct compression technique. Each superdisintegrant is used in 3 different increased concentrations. The pre compression parameters of the prepared tablet blend like angle of repose, bulk density, tapped density, Carr's index, and Hausner's ratio were determined. Post compression parameters for prepared tablet formulations like hardness, friability, weight variation, in vitro dispersion time and in vitro disintegration time were evaluated. Formulation (F9) with 6 mg croscarmellose sodium shows low disintegration time. The optimized formulation F9 was found to be complying with all the properties of tablets.

Keywords: *Fast disintegrating tablets, Diclofenac sodium, Croscarmellose sodium, crospovidone, sodium starch glycolate*

Presented as Oral Presentation

Formulation Development And *In-vitro* Evaluation Of Fast Dissolving Oral Films Of Domperidone Employing Super Disintegrants

Scan to View online

Presented by
Dr. Venkateswarlu Kudipudi
Aditya College of Pharmacy, Aditya University, Surampalem, Andhra Pradesh, India

Abstract

Recently, fast dissolving drug delivery system have started gaining popularity and acceptance as new drug delivery systems, because they are easy to administer and lead to better compliance. Fast-dissolving oral delivery systems are solid dosage forms, which disintegrate or dissolve within 1 min when placed in the mouth without drinking or chewing. Sodium carboxy methyl cellulose, polyvinyl alcohol, sodium alginate were selected as polymers, after pre-formulation studies polyvinyl alcohol selected as a best film polymer for domperidone films, Glycerine as plasticizers, aspartame as sweetener and, anhydrous banana powder and sodium starch glycolate are used as a super disintigrants. The prepared films were evaluated further by different characterisation tests. Formulation was developed based on polymer concentration and super disintegrants in the concentration of 0.5:0.5% and 1:1% of anhydrous banana powder and sodium starch glycolate are crucial for low disintegration time. The prepared films are evaluated for thickness, weight variation, assay, surface pH, folding endurance, swelling index, disintegration time, *in-vitro* dissolution, release order kinetics (zero order and first order) were applied for optimized formulation F5, F6, F11 and, F12. Acceptable properties were obtained in the batch F5, F6, F11 and, F12 the *in-vitro* disintegration time was below 30 seconds. It was concluded that formulations F5, F6, F11 and, F 12 were found to be satisfactory batches and were optimized for the desirable properties.

Keywords: *Domperidone, Fast dissolving, Super disintigrants, Banana powder, Sodium starch glycolate, combined polymers*

Presented as Oral Presentation

Bionic Eye – Visual Prosthesis

Scan to View online

Presented by
Dr. Boddeda Benarjee Veera Mani Kishore
Vignan Institute of Pharmaceutical Technology, Visakhapatnam, Andhra Pradesh, India

Abstract

Bionic eye is an artificial electronic eye which provokes visual sensations in the brain by directly stimulating different parts of the optic nerve. The main purpose of bionic eye is to provide vision, partially to the visually challenged people by the use of modern-day electronic devices like charge coupled device (CCD) camera and bionic eye implant. The implant is a small chip that is surgically implanted behind the retina in the eye ball. However, it presents a novel idea of integrating a new approach of bionic eye with the nanogenerator. The nanogenerator is multifaced when compared to the external batteries providing better power, compactness and higher efficiency. Bionic eye represent a promising and rapidly advancing technology with the potential to restore vision and improve the quality of life for individuals with visual impairments. As the field continues to evolve, we can anticipate even greater breakthroughs in visual prosthetics, offering hope to countless individuals seeking to regain their sight.

Keywords: *Bionic eye, charge coupled device camera, bionic eye implant, retinal prosthesis*

Presented as Oral Presentation

CRISPR CAS9: Targeted Genome Editing And How It Can Change Our Future

Scan to View online

Presented by
Dr. P Aditi Naidu
Vignan Institute of Pharmaceutical Technology, Visakhapatnam, Andhra Pradesh, India

Abstract

The first observation of CRISPR clustered repeats were discovered by ishino in 1987. The first human CRISPR/CAS 9 trial was made in 2016. CRISPR are sections of genetic code containing short repetition of base sequences followed by spaces DNA segments CRISPR is a revolutionary technique modified any region of the genome of that can be any species with high precision and accuracy without harming other genes. Formation of editing complex, pairing with the target gene, cutting the target DNA, inserting a new gene, production of the desired product. Significance: deleting of gene, adding a gene, activation of dead gene, control gene activation. Conclusion: Scientists are experimenting with using CRISPR to engineer "gene drives" to spread specific genes through a population of insect pests that cause them to die or become infertile. Researchers are looking to CRISPR CAS9 as a technique for editing out genetic defects that result in sickle cell disease, cystic fibrosis, for developing more targeted and effective cancer treatment.

Keywords: CRISPR CAS9, Target Genome editing,gene drives

Presented as Oral Presentation

Nanoparticle-Based Antivenoms: A Novel Approach To Counter Snakebite Envenoming - A Review

Scan to View online

Presented by
Miss Sanipini Sri Lakshmi
Aditya College of Pharmacy, Aditya University, Surampalem, Andhra Pradesh, India

Abstract

Snakebite envenomation is a significant public health issue, responsible for numerous deaths and severe morbidity. The World Health Organization (WHO) has categorized it as a neglected tropical disease. This problem is particularly severe in rural India, where four major venomous snakes—the common cobra (Naja naja), common krait (Bungarus caeruleus), Russell's viper (Daboia russelii), and saw-scaled viper (Echis carinatus)—are the primary culprits behind most snakebite cases. Globally, snakebites affect approximately 2.5 million people annually, resulting in around 100,000 deaths, with India alone reporting 15,000 fatalities. This review highlights the potential of various nanoparticles (NPs), including hydrogel nanoparticles, Titanium dioxide NPs (TiO2-NPs), gold NPs (AuNP) conjugated with 2-hydroxy-4-methoxy benzoic acid (HMBA), Vitex negundo-conjugated gold NPs (VN-AuNP), Curcumin-conjugated gold NPs (C-GNP), silver NPs (AgNPs) synthesized from Dryopteris cochleate rhizomes, and alginic acid-based AgNPs, in neutralizing snake venom. These nanoparticles have demonstrated potential in preventing tissue damage, toxin spread, and organ toxicity. Further research is essential to explore the full potential of nanoparticles in treating snakebites and addressing the limitations of current antivenom therapies. If successful, nanoparticle-based treatments could revolutionize snakebite management, especially in resource-limited areas where access to ASV is scarce.

Keywords: *ASV, anti snake venom, nanoparticles, gold based nanoparticles, silver based nanoparticles, venomous snakes*

Presented as Oral Presentation

The Future Of Pharmacogenomics In Personalized Medicine

Scan to View online

Presented by
Mr. Madduri Sivamani
Aditya Pharmacy College, Aditya University, Surampalem, Andhra Pradesh, India

Abstract

Pharmacogenomics is revolutionizing personalized medicine by tailoring treatments to an inividual's genetic makeup. This talk explores how pharmacogenomics can improve treatment quality and reduce adverse drug reactions by tailoring medication plans to a patient's unique history. We'll cover the basic principles of pharmacogenomics and review key studies that demonstrate its therapeutic efficacy across a variety of conditions, demonstrating its ability to improve patient outcomes. We'll also discuss the challenges clinicians face in integrating pharmacogenomics into daily practice, including interventions that impact business, ethics, and education. It's important for clinicians to ensure they can use this information effectively in patient care. Finally, we'll look at the future of pharmacogenomics in drug development and its role in personalized medicine. gender paves the way for greater pharmacogenomics Effective, personalized treatment strategies can benefit patients.

Keywords: *Pharmacogenomics, Personalized medicine, Treatment quality, Adverse drug reactions, Patient outcomes, Drug development*

Presented as Oral Presentation

Formulation And *In-vitro* Evaluation Of Atorvastatin Calcium Liquisolid Tablets

Scan to View online

Presented by
Dr. Madhavi Latha Samala
Aditya College of Pharmacy, Aditya University, Surampalem, Andhra Pradesh, India

Abstract

The study's major goal was to develop and test atorvastatin calcium (ATC) liquisolid tablets with various excipient ratios to improve aqueous solubility and thereby increase bioavailability.

Three distinct liquisolid formulations F1, F2, and F3 of atorvasatin calcium (ATC) were created utilizing three different excipient ratios (5, 10, and 15) at a fixed liquid vehicle concentration of 20% w/w. Carrier and coating polymer concentrations were estimated using the excipient ratios and associated formulae. All formulations were examined for their pre-compression, post-compression, and *in-vitro* dissolving capabilities. The produced mixes for liquisolid tablets demonstrated good flow characteristics. The thickness of the compacted tablets ranged from 3.20 to 3.34 mm, with a hardness of 4.14 to 4.32 kg/sq.cm. When compared to other formulations, F1 demonstrated faster and more complete drug release within 60 minutes. The best formulation, F1, was compared to the standard directly compressed tablet formulation, F4.

The findings of the study indicate that liquisolid formulation techniques have promising potential for the development of immediate and rapid drug release dosage forms.

Keywords: *Liquisolid systems, Atorvastatin Calcium (ATC), Solubility enhancement, flowability, drug release*

Presented as Oral Presentation

Phytosomal Drug Delivery Systems

Scan to View online

Presented by
Dr. Sailaja Gunnam
Gokaraju Rangaraju College of Pharmacy,
Hyderabad, Telangana, India

Abstract

Phytosomal drug delivery systems have emerged as a novel approach to overcoming the limitations associated with the bioavailability and efficacy of phytochemicals. Phytochemicals, including flavonoids, terpenoids, alkaloids, and polyphenols, are known for their therapeutic potential in various disease conditions. However, their clinical application is often limited due to poor water solubility, instability, and low bioavailability. Phytosomes, which form a lipid-compatible molecular complex between phytochemicals and phospholipids, have been shown to significantly improve the absorption, stability, and bioavailability of these bioactive compounds. This review provides a comprehensive analysis of the advancements in phytosomal drug delivery systems, focusing on their formulation techniques, physicochemical properties, mechanisms of enhanced absorption, various preparation methods and there characterization. Furthermore, the review explores the therapeutic applications of phytosomes in the treatment of chronic diseases, such as cancer, cardiovascular diseases, inflammation, and liver disorders. Phytosomal drug delivery offers a promising avenue for enhancing the pharmacokinetic profiles of phytochemicals, improving their therapeutic potential.

Keywords: *Phytosomes, Phytochemicals, Drug Delivery, Bioavailability, Therapeutic Applications*

Presented as Oral Presentation

In -Vitro Pharmacological Evaluation Of Fresh Leaf Decoction Of Psidium Guajava(Linn.) And Murraya Koenigii (Linn.) Spreng

Scan to View online

Presented by
Miss P. Santhi
VV Institute of Pharmaceutical Sciences,
Gudlavalleru, Andhra Pradesh, India

Abstract

The increasing prevalence of maladaptive dietary habits has become a primary factor driving the rise of Diabetes mellitus—a hallmark disease of modern civilization. This chronic condition and its associated comorbidities, such as diabetic nephropathy, retinopathy, and neuropathy, impose significant health and economic burdens, ultimately diminishing the quality of life. Complementary and alternative medicine suggests that certain herbs may offer safe and effective therapeutic options, proposing them as gentle, natural alternatives to conventional medicine. Among these, Psidium guajava (guava) and Murraya koenigii (curry leaf) are reputed for their extensive applications in traditional medicinal systems, especially in treating respiratory ailments. Given this background, a systematic investigation of Psidium guajava and Murraya koenigii using established traditional drug screening methods may help translate the concept of dietary management of metabolic disorders into practical reality. This study aims to explore the pharmacological potential of these plants, providing foundational insights for the development of plant-based formulations that could complement modern therapeutic approaches to diabetes management.

Keywords: *Diabetes mellitus, maladaptive diet, diabetic nephropathy, diabetic retinopathy, diabetic neuropathy, complementary medicine, alternative medicine, Psidium guajava,Murraya koenigii*

Presented as Oral Presentation

Computational Tools In Drug Discovery

Scan to View online

Presented by
Dr. Naga Bharathi.Marni
Vignan Institute of Pharmaceutical Technology, Visakhapatnam, Andhra Pradesh, India

Abstract

The drug discovery process has been significantly transformed through the integration of computational tools, which enhance the speed and precision of identifying viable therapeutic candidates. This systematic review offers a comprehensive overview of key computational methodologies used in drug discovery, including molecular docking, quantitative structure-activity relationship (QSAR) modeling, virtual screening, molecular dynamics simulations, and machine learning techniques. A systematic search was performed across multiple databases, including PubMed, Scopus, Web of Science, and Google Scholar, to identify relevant articles published between 2010 and 2023. The search terms included "computational tools in drug discovery," "molecular docking," "QSAR modeling," "virtual screening," "molecular dynamics," and "machine learning in pharmacology." Inclusion criteria focused on studies that emphasized computational methodologies, provided empirical data or case studies, and were published in peer-reviewed journals, while excluding reviews and studies lacking robust methodologies. The findings reveal that while computational tools have significantly advanced drug discovery, challenges in effective integration and data quality persist. Interdisciplinary collaboration among chemists, biologists, and data scientists is crucial for overcoming these challenges and maximizing the potential of computational approaches, ultimately streamlining the drug development process.

Keywords: *Drug Discovery, Molecular Docking, Computational Tools*

Presented as Oral Presentation

Ameliorative Action Of Passiflora Foetida On Non-Alcoholic Fatty Liver Disease: A Holistic Approach

Scan to View online

Presented by
Dr. P. Veeresh Babu
Gokaraju Rangaraju College of Pharmacy,
Hyderabad, Telangana, India

Abstract

Non-alcoholic fatty liver disease (NAFLD) is the most common liver disease worldwide and the leading cause of liver-related morbidity and mortality. NAFLD is a condition caused by accumulation or build-up of fats in liver which is not due to heavy consumption of alcohol. The present study aims to evaluate the beneficial role of methanolic extract of Passiflora foetida in NAFLD. The GC–MS analysis of methanolic extract of Passiflora foetida detected the presence of 11 phytochemical compounds. The extract also showed prominent pancreatic lipase inhibitory activity and the IC50 value was comparable to that of the standard orlistat. HFHCC diet was used to induce NAFLD in mice, and the disease induced mice were treated with methanolic extract of Passiflora foetida at 200 and 400 mg/kg. The reduced levels of TC, TG, LDL, VLDL, AST and ALT and elevated levels of HDL in treatment groups demonstrated its anti-NAFLD potency and the effect of extract at 400mg/kg was comparable to that of the pioglitazone. In tetracycline induced NAFLD, extract significantly decreased TC, TG, LDL, VLDL, AST and ALT levels and elevated levels of HDL substantiating its anti-NAFLD potency. Histopathological examination of liver cells further corroborated the results obtained from the *in vivo* models. The study revealed the beneficial role of Passiflora foetida in non-alcoholic fatty liver disease which can be attributed to flavonoids, phenols, alkaloids present in the extract.

Keywords: *Passiflora foetida, NAFLD, HFHCC diet, Tetracycline, Flavonoids, Alkaloids*

Presented as Oral Presentation

Formulation And Evaluation Of Amlodipine Sustained Release Microspheres

Scan to View online

Presented by
Mrs. Prasanthi Teella
Aditya College of Pharmacy, Aditya University, Surampalem, Andhra Pradesh, India

Abstract

In the present study we prepared amlodipine microspheres which is having long lasting effect without any side effects caused by immediate release dosage forms. Amlodipine microspheres are prepared by using sodium alginate polymers with different ratio. All microspheres were incorporated into pre and post compression studies. All the studies showed the results with Indian pharmacopoeia limits. In the present study we prepared Amlodipine sustained release microspheres. Which is having long lasting effect with out any side effects caused by immediate release dosage forms. Amlodipine microspheres are prepared by using Sodium alginate, hydroxy propyl methyl cellulose, Carbopol polymers with different ratios. By using Sodium alginate polymer F1,F2,F3 formulations were prepared. F4, F5, F6 formulations are prepared by Hydroxy Methyl cellulose. F7, F8, F9 formulations are prepared by Carbopol. All the microspheres were incorporated into pre and post compression studies (Bulk density, Tapped density, Hausner's ratio, Carr's index. All showed the results within the IP limits. Out of all the formulations F2 shows the best release.

Keywords: *Amlodipine, Microspheres, Compression studies, Immediate release dosage forms, Hydroxy Methyl cellulose*

Presented as Oral Presentation

A Novel Strategy To Enhance Its Bioavailability For The Management Of Hyperlipidemia

Scan to View online

Presented by
Mrs. Mohammad Bakhatwar
Gokaraju Rangaraju College of Pharmacy,
Hyderabad, Telangana, India

Abstract

Hyperlipidemia, a metabolic condition marked by elevated plasma levels of cholesterol or triglyceride-carrying lipoproteins, is a major contributor to atherosclerosis and cardiovascular diseases. Antihyperlipidemic drugs are classified according to their primary mechanism of action. Fenofibrate's role in regulating cholesterol and managing insulin resistance-associated metabolic disorders makes it a preferred choice in combination therapies with statins for cardiovascular disease management. Nanoparticles have gained attention for enhancing the bioavailability of poorly water-soluble drugs by reducing particle size to the nanoscale (100-200 nm), which increases solubility, dissolution rate, and adhesion to cell surfaces. Nanosuspensions improve drug solubility and bioavailability through methods like media milling, high-pressure homogenization, and precipitation. Despite advancements, producing stable Fenofibrate nanoparticles below 100 nm at an industrial scale remains a challenge. Recent strategies include using sonication and freeze-drying to enhance bioavailability and solubility, achieving significant improvements in drug dissolution and therapeutic efficacy.

Keywords: *Fenofibrate, Nanoparticles, Bioavailability, Nanosuspension, Solubility, High pressure homogenization.*

Presented as Oral Presentation

Nanohybrids - A Brief Review And Its Applications

Scan to View online

Presented by
Mr. Kancharla Kameswararao
University College of Pharmaceutical sciences, Acharya Nagarjuna University, Namburu, Andhra Pradesh, India

Abstract

Nanotechnology is a branch of science devoted to producing and using structures, devices & systems by manipulating atoms and molecules at the nanoscale, to a great extent in the last decades. It has several sizes, shapes, colours, and materials improving mechanical strength, thermal stability, optical properties, electrical conductivity, biocompatibility, customizable surface chemistry, and sustainability. Nanohybrids are classified into different types based on their parent material, the material used for nanohybrids, and the interaction between the two phases. Nanohybrids have a wide range of applications in various fields including photocatalysis, energy storage, designing of drug delivery systems for diagnosis treatment, enhanced bioavailability, and masking the bitter taste and fuel cells as a catalyst. Nanohybrids act as contrast agents for imaging like MRI, CT, X-ray, IR, NIR, and phototherapy & photodynamic therapy. Nanohybrids also play an important role in pandemic conditions to control and prevent transmission of virus to prepare of PPE, air filter masks & biomedical waste management. Nanohybrids are also helpful as mosquito larvicides and are also used in biomedical devices. Nanohybrids also have wound-healing properties by promoting tissue regeneration, improving tissue strength and elasticity. This review mainly focuses on nanohybrid characters, types and applications in various fields.

Keywords: *Nanohybrids, Hybrid materials, Nanotechnology, Nanoparticulates.*

Presented as Oral Presentation

Advanced Nanotechnolgy Methods For The Analytical Characterisation And Monitoring Of Abraxane

Scan to View online

Presented by
Miss Sree Geetha Adathakula
Aditya College of Pharmacy, Aditya University, Surampalem, Andhra Pradesh, India

Abstract

Abraxane a nanoparticle-bound formulation of Paclitaxel,has emerged as a breakthrough in cancer therapy due to its enhanced drug delivery,solubility,and reduced toxicity.The complex nature of Abraxane's nanoparticles necessitates the use of advanced analytical techniques for its characterisation and evaluation.The present research focusses on application of nanotechnology based methods to analyse and monitor. The research also explores the role of nanotechnolgy in assessing the biodistribution and drug release profiles of Abraxane, providing critical data for optimizing its therapeutic efficacy, optimizing the dosing and minimising the side effects. In conclusion nanotechnology driven analytical techniques are crucial for the detailed characterisation and evaluation of Abraxane in pharmaceutical applications.These methods not only improve drug formulation analysis but also contribute to the development of more effective and personalised cancer treatment strategies,reinforcing the importance of nanotechnology in modern drug development and therapeutic monitoring.Moreover these methods are used to study that nanomaterials can be engineered to interact with specific drug molecules for their real time monitoring .

Keywords: *Abraxane, paclitaxel, Nanotechnolgy,sensitvity,therapeutic drug monitoring,nanosensors etc.*

Presented as Oral Presentation

Surveying Physical Literacy In 10-15 Year-Olds: A Gender-Based Comparative Study In Kakinada

Scan to View online

Presented by
Dr. Pavan Kumar Yanamadala
Aditya Pharmacy College, Aditya University, Surampalem, Andhra Pradesh, India

Abstract

Physical literacy encompasses a person's capacity to participate in physical activities with assurance and skill over the course of their life. A six-month cross-sectional survey involved 220 students (112 males and 108 females) from various schools in Kakinada, India. Participants were assessed using the Canadian Assessment of Physical Literacy-2 scale, covering four domains: daily behaviour, physical competence, knowledge and understanding, and motivation and confidence. The sample was randomly selected, and data were collected using a pedometer and a questionnaire. The findings showed that physical literacy rates were 76.12% for boys and 68.31% for girls. Boys outperformed girls in all areas except knowledge and understanding, which were the weakest for both genders (59.34% for boys, and 52.57% for girls). In daily behaviour and physical competence, boys scored 68.14% while girls scored 71.19%. Girls also demonstrated lower engagement in physical activities due to social, environmental, and biological factors. The research found that while boys generally showed higher physical literacy, girls faced significant disadvantages in knowledge and comprehension. To improve physical literacy among girls, targeted interventions are needed to address these gaps. Additionally, addressing societal and environmental barriers can help reduce the gender divide and promote more active lifestyles for all children.

Keywords: *Physical literacy, School children, Gender differences, Physical competence, Motivation, Knowledge*

Presented as Oral Presentation

Formulation And Evaluation Of Antiviral Drug Sofosbuvir Microspheres For Capsule System

Scan to View online

Presented by
Dr. S Satyalakshmi
Vignan Institute of Pharmaceutical Technology, Visakhapatnam, Andhra Pradesh, India

Abstract

This study aimed to develop and evaluate a microencapsulated sofosbuvir formulation for delivery within a capsule. For this purpose, the emulsion solvent evaporation method was used. An organic phase, comprising a volatile solvent, a dissolved polymer (HPMC) and an encapsulated drug, forms an emulsion which is subsequently emulsified in an aqueous phase. HPMC as the polymer retards drug release, while ethyl cellulose facilitates controlled drug release. Through SEM imaging, the microscopic size and shape of the particles were evaluated. The yields of all formulations (F1-F6) varied between 76.41% and 81.63%. Formulation F3 showed the highest entrapment efficiency at 78.55% while the overall efficiency ranged between 69.67% and 78.55%. Flow properties and other characteristics of the material were evaluated through pre-compression studies. F3 released 90.45% of the drug within 12 hours. The SEM images revealed uniform and spherical microspheres from the optimized formulation. According to the Higuchi model, the optimized formulation exhibited zero-order release kinetics with non-Fickian diffusion behavior. The optimized formulation exhibited suitable flow properties, as established through assessments, for capsule filling, while the resulting capsules passed official specifications. The use of the specific polymer significantly enhanced the microspheres' flow properties and facilitated the prolonged release of sofosbuvir.

Keywords: *Microspheres, Sofosbuvir, Capsule, Controlled release, Anti-viral drug*

Presented as Oral Presentation

Study On Women With The Polycystic Ovary Syndrome And Their Health Related Quality Of Life

Scan to View online

Presented by
Miss Velisetti Kranthi Swaroopa
Aditya College of Pharmacy, Aditya University, Surampalem, Andhra Pradesh, India

Abstract

Polycystic Ovary Syndrome (PCOS) is a hormonal disorder affecting 4-12% of reproductive-aged women, leading to menstrual irregularities, hyperandrogenism, and metabolic complications. Objective: To assess the health-related quality of life (HRQOL) in women with PCOS and explore its correlation with clinical manifestations, treatment outcomes, and emotional well-being. A prospective observational study was conducted at GSL General Hospital and Medical College, Rajahmundry, involving 100 PCOS patients diagnosed using Rotterdam criteria. Data was collected through questionnaires, patient case sheets, and laboratory tests. The study revealed significant impacts on HRQOL, including emotional struggles (56%), irregular menstruation (87%), hirsutism (18%), and weight concerns (64%). Treatment regimens, including metformin and hormonal contraceptives, improved symptoms and quality of life. Our findings correlate with existing literature highlighting PCOS's negative impact on HRQOL, particularly emotional well-being. Early diagnosis, comprehensive treatment, and emotional support are crucial for improving quality of life in PCOS patients. Conclusion:PCOS significantly affects women's physical and emotional health. Multidisciplinary management strategies and support systems are essential to enhance HRQOL and mitigate long-term health risks.

Keywords: *Polycystic Ovary Syndrome, Health-Related Quality of Life, Hormonal Imbalance, Menstrual Irregularities, Hyperandrogenism, Metabolic Complications.*

Presented as Oral Presentation

Improving The Penetration Ability Of Poorly Permeable Drug By Vesicular Drug Delivery System- Cubosomes

Scan to View online

Presented by
Mrs. Sesha Sai Durga Manyam
Aditya College of Pharmacy, Aditya University, Surampalem, Andhra Pradesh, India

Abstract

The objective of present research work is aimed to enhance the permeability of poorly permeable class –III drug like fexofenadine HCl. cubosomes are novel lipid based vesicular drug delivery systems similar to liposomes and niosomes. In the present study glyceryl mono oleate was selected as a lipid and pluronics -127 was taken in three different ratios to formulate various formulations (F1,F2,F3) of cubosomes loaded with drug fexofenadine HCl. Three different formulations of cubosomes were prepared by top-down method. all formulations were characterized for various evaluation studies like particle size , zeta potential, entrapement efficiency, *In vivo* drug release studies. From the above evaluation studies the optimized formulation was selected. Ex-vivo skin permeation studies were carried out for the optimized formulation. From the results of all the evaluation studies and ex-vivo skin permeation studies it was concluded that cubosomes are the promising technique for enhancing the permeation of class- III drugs like fexofenadine.

Keywords: *cubosomes, vesicular drud delivery,glyceryl monosterate, fexofenaidne*

Presented as Oral Presentation

Antibiotics: A Medical Revolution Under Threat From Resistance.

Scan to View online

Presented by
Miss A.B.S.D. Padma Sri
Aditya College of Pharmacy, Aditya University, Surampalem, Andhra Pradesh, India

Abstract

Since their discovery in the early 20th century, antibiotics have transformed medicine, saving millions of lives by effectively treating bacterial infections. However, this progress is now at risk due to the alarming rise of antibiotic resistance. The misuse and overuse of these drugs, combined with the remarkable adaptability of bacteria, have accelerated the development of resistant strains, creating a significant global health challenge. This article traces the origins of antibiotics and examines how bacterial resistance has emerged and evolved. The rise of resistant infections carries serious consequences—longer hospital stays, increased mortality rates, and soaring healthcare costs. It is estimated that antibiotic-resistant infections already cause around 700,000 deaths annually, with this number projected to rise unless urgent action is taken. Tackling this crisis requires a multifaceted approach. Drug repurposing—identifying new uses for existing drugs—offers a practical and cost-efficient avenue to accelerate the development of new treatments. Simultaneously, discovering novel drug targets and refining current therapies can strengthen the fight against resistance. This review underscores the need for robust research, global collaboration, and innovative solutions to restrain antibiotic resistance and protect public health for future generation.

Keywords: *Antibiotic resistance, novel drug targets, innovative solution.*

Presented as Oral Presentation

Applicability Of Tragacanth In The Design Of Hydrochlorothiazide Floating Tablets

Scan to View online

Presented by
Dr. J. Anu Pravallika
Aditya College of Pharmacy, Aditya University, Surampalem, Andhra Pradesh, India

Abstract

The creation of oral sustained-controlled release formulations aims to gradually release the drug in the gastrointestinal tract, ensuring a sustained and effective drug concentration in the systemic circulation over a prolonged duration. Hydrochlorothiazide is a thiazide-type diuretic with short half-life selected as model drug for this study. The main aim of the present study was to evaluate the applicability of tragacanth (natural polymer) in the design of gastric floating tablets of hydrochlorothiazide by direct compression method and the efficiency of this polymer is compared with already established synthetic polymer, carbopol 934. The prepared tablets underwent evaluation for drug and excipients compatibility using FTIR studies, precompression and post compression parameters, buoyancy studies and *in-vitro* drug release studies. The FTIR analysis revealed no evidence of physical or chemical interaction between the drug and excipients. The precompression parameters were deemed suitable for formulation development, and post compression parameters were found to be within acceptable limits and satisfactory. Among all the formulations prepared with tragacanth, 1:1.75 drug : polymer ratio (HZT5) exhibited sustained release over a period of 6 hours when compared with synthetic polymer carbopol 934 with the same ratio. Hence, these gastric floating systems containing tragacanth polymer may be a valuable alternative over the conventional systems.

Keywords: *Gastric floating tablets, hydrochlorothiazide, tragacanth, carbopol 934, direct compression method.*

Presented as Oral Presentation

Pharmacological Evaluation Of A Plant Extract Against Scopolamine Induced Dementia Of Alzheimer's Type In Wistar Rats

Scan to View online

Presented by
K.V. NagaLakshmi
VJs College of Pharmacy

Abstract

One of the most common cause of dementia is Alzheimer's disease. The word dementia includes a symptoms like memory loss, difficulties in thinking, problem-solving or language, decrease in social activity. None of the treatments available today for Alzheimer's disease stops the malfunction and death of neurons in the brain that cause Alzheimer's symptoms. In traditional use of medicine, many plants are available to treat the symptoms of Alzheimer's. Grass extract which belongs to family of Poacea, is proved for having anti anxiety, anti oxidant, anti inflammatory etc. The present study was designed to evaluate the protective effect of Plant extract against Scopolamine induced Alzheimer's type dementia in Albino wistar rats. Alzheimers type dementia was screened by observing behavioural parameters using actophotometer (locomotory activity), morris Water Maze (spatial learning), y maze (exploratory behaviour) and biochemical estimations such as catalase, glutathione, acetyl cholinesterase, malondialdehyde. The plant extract has shown that the decrease in the symptoms of Alzheimer's type dementia by ameliorating locomotory activity, spatial learning, exploratory behaviour and increased antioxidant enzyme levels in the brain

Keywords: *Actophotometer, Morris water maze, Y maze, Catalase, Acetyl cholinesterase, Glutathione, Malondialdehyde*

Presented as Oral Presentation

Formulation And Characterisation Of Mucoadhesive Buccal Films By Employing Natural Polymers

Scan to View online

Presented by
Mrs. Arumilli Swetha
Aditya College of Pharmacy, Aditya University, Surampalem, Andhra Pradesh, India

Abstract

Buccal drug delivery systems present a prospective avenue for the administration of drugs to the buccal mucosa for the treatment of oral diseases, as well as for systemic distribution through mucosal absorption into the systemic circulation at a regulated and preset rate. Therapeutic drugs are absorbed through the oral mucosa, which increases systemic bioavailability by preventing active drug loss from first-pass hepatic metabolism and early drug breakdown caused by gastrointestinal tract pH and enzyme activity and it provides effective therapy to patient groups unable to swallow or with swallowing difficulties. Additionally, unlike the sublingual route and tablets the buccal mucosa allows a prolonged retention of a dose form, particularly with the application of mucoadhesive polymers and of multiple layers of the dosage form, without greatly interfering with functions like speech or mastication. Natural polymers have recently gained importance in pharmaceutical field by enhancing the dosage form's contact time and residence time with the mucous membrane. Buccal films can be formulated by using natural polymers like sodium alginate, guar gum, tragacanth, karaya gum, gelatin, pectin, chitosan. Films can be prepared by solvent casting method, hot melt extrusion, inkjet printing and three-dimensional printing. Buccal films should be characterised for physical appearance, Thickness, Swelling index, folding endurance, surface PH, percentage moisture absorption, mucoadhesive strength and invitro drug release studies.

Keywords: *Buccal films, first-pass effect, Natural Polymers, mucous membrane, Characteristion.*

Presented as Oral Presentation

Advanced Hyphenated Analytical Techniques For Modern Pharmaceutical Analysis And Quality Control

Scan to View online

Presented by
Mrs. Vinny Therissa Mangam
Aditya College of Pharmacy, Aditya University, Surampalem, Andhra Pradesh, India

Abstract

Hyphenated analytical techniques have revolutionized pharmaceutical analysis by combining the separating power of chromatography with the identification capabilities of spectroscopic methods. Modern developments in LC-MS/MS technology offer enhanced sensitivity and selectivity for complex pharmaceutical matrices, facilitating simultaneous analysis of multiple components. The implementation of two-dimensional liquid chromatography (2D-LC) coupled with mass spectrometry has addressed the challenges of analyzing complex pharmaceutical formulations and biological samples. Advanced data processing algorithms and artificial intelligence integration have enhanced the interpretation of complex spectral data. These hyphenated techniques have found extensive applications in drug development, stability studies, metabolite identification, and quality control processes. The combination of chromatographic separation with multiple detection systems has become indispensable in meeting regulatory requirements for pharmaceutical analysis. Continuous improvements in instrument design, automation, and data processing capabilities are driving the evolution of hyphenated techniques toward greater accuracy, sensitivity, and throughput in pharmaceutical analysis.

Keywords: *Hyphenated techniques, Mass spectrometry, Chromatography coupling, Pharmaceutical analysis, Spectroscopic detection*

Presented as Oral Presentation

Development And Validation Of Uplc Method For Simultaneous Determination Of Emtricitabine And Efavirenz In Tablet Dosage Form

Scan to View online

Presented by
Miss Kruthiventi Sai Priyanka
Aditya College of Pharmacy, Aditya University, Surampalem, Andhra Pradesh, India

Abstract

A new, simple, sensitive, accurate, reproducible ,reliable analytical method was developed and validated for simultaneous estimation of emtricitabine and efavirenz in tablet dosage form by using UPLC method. The separation is achieved by Grace Smart C18 (4.6 X 50mm,1.7μm) column. Methanol and potassium dihydrogen orthophosphate buffer in ratio of 65:35 at a flow rate of 0.3ml/min. the column is maintained at ambient temperature. Both the drugs measured at 260nm. Run time is maintained for 5 mins. Linearity lies from 10-50 μg/ml for emtricitabine and 20-100 μg/ml for efavirenz. The method was validated for system suitability, precision , accuracy, specificity, ruggedness, robustness, LOD, LOQ were found within the limits. % recovery ranges from 98%-102% for emtricitabine and efavirenz. Hence it is concluded that the proposed method was good approach for obtaining reliable results and found to be suitable for routine analysis.

Keywords: *UPLC,emtricitabine,efavirenz,potassium dihydrogen orthophosphate buffer,system suitability,*

Presented as Oral Presentation

Nosocomial Infections And Antimicrobial Resistance: An Evaluation From A Tertiary Care Hospital In Kakinada

Scan to View online

Presented by
Miss Hepzibah Rani Gidla
Aditya Pharmacy College, Aditya University, Surampalem, Andhra Pradesh, India

Abstract

The increasing incidence of nosocomial infections (NIs) presents significant challenges within the healthcare sector, particularly in light of the escalating issue of antimicrobial resistance (AMR). A retrospective cross-sectional study spanning six months (March-September 2024) was performed, involving patients diagnosed with NIs. Out of 310 samples, UTIs were the most frequently observed (47.83%), followed by Sepsis (38.47%) and Pneumonia (18.54%). Gram-negative bacteria were predominant (65.25%), with Citrobacter spp. (31.54%), Escherichia coli (29.54%), and Klebsiella spp. (15.67%) identified as the leading pathogens. Among Gram-positive bacteria, Enterococcus spp. was the most common (15.54%), while methicillin-resistant Staphylococcus aureus (MRSA) and vancomycin-resistant Enterococcus (VRE) were found at rates of 15.87% and 65.14%, respectively. Notably, carbapenem resistance was detected in 65.9% of Citrobacter spp., 47.3% of E. coli, and 41.45% of Klebsiella spp., with 3.88% of Citrobacter spp. and 24% of Klebsiella spp. classified as extensively drug-resistant (XDR). The significant prevalence of carbapenem-resistant Enterobacteriaceae and the high rates of VRE highlight the urgent necessity for rigorous antibiotic stewardship and improved infection control strategies to mitigate the proliferation of resistant pathogens.

Keywords: *Antimicrobial resistance, nosocomial infections, Gram-negative bacteria, VRE, MRSA, Carbapenem-resistant bacteria.*

Presented as Oral Presentation

Design And Insilico Screening Of Azitidinone And Thiazolidinone Hybrids Of Niacin Hydrazide For Anti-Tubercular And Anti-Cancer Activities.

Scan to View online

Presented by
Dr. Ponnam Chiranjeevi
Vignan Institute of Pharmaceutical Technology, Visakhapatnam, Andhra Pradesh, India

Abstract

The present research involves design and insilico screening of azitidinone and thiazolidinone hybrids of niacin hydrazide for their potential anti-tubercular and anti-cancer activities. All the twelve ligands showed better binding score then the drug Imepenam (IMP) taken for comparison in insilico screening for Anti-tubercular activity. Eleven ligands except the ligand TH01(Thiazolidine derivative without any substitution) have shown better binding energies then the drug Erlotinib(ETB) taken as standard for comparison in insilico screening against for anti-cancer activity. One ligand have three common amino acids GLN A:317, ALA A:99, LEU A:316 in protein 3UPN interacting with drug imipenem. Similarly six ligands have more than three common amino acids each in the protein structure 4HJO interacting with the drug erlotinib suggesting that these ligands would have same mechanism of action as that of erlotinib, five ligands have binding score more than the standard drug Erlotinib. Future work may involve synthesizing and testing the selected candidates invitro and invivo to validate their efficacy and safety profiles. This approach offers a cost-effective and efficient strategy for prioritizing compounds for further experimental validation, thereby accelerating drug discovery efforts in combating these significant global health challenges.

Keywords: *Azitidinone, Thiazolidinone, Anti-cancer Activity, Anti-tubercular Activity, 4HJO, 3UPN, Molecular Docking*

Presented as Oral Presentation

Study On Women With The Polycystic Ovary Syndrome And Their Health Related Quality Of Life By Confirmatory Analysis In A Tertiary Care Hospital

Scan to View online

Presented by
Miss Velisetti Kranthi Swaroopa
Aditya College of Pharmacy, Aditya University, Surampalem, Andhra Pradesh, India

Abstract

Polycystic Ovary Syndrome (PCOS) is a hormonal disorder affecting 4-12% of reproductive-aged women, leading to menstrual irregularities, hyperandrogenism, and metabolic complications. To assess the health-related quality of life (HRQOL) in women with PCOS and explore its correlation with clinical manifestations, treatment outcomes, and emotional well-being. Methods: A prospective observational study was conducted at GSL General Hospital and Medical College, Rajahmundry, involving 100 PCOS patients diagnosed using Rotterdam criteria. Data was collected through questionnaires, patient case sheets, and laboratory tests. Results:The study revealed significant impacts on HRQOL, including emotional struggles (56%), irregular menstruation (87%), hirsutism (18%), and weight concerns (64%). Treatment regimens, including metformin and hormonal contraceptives, improved symptoms and quality of life. Our findings correlate with existing literature highlighting PCOS's negative impact on HRQOL, particularly emotional well-being. Early diagnosis, comprehensive treatment, and emotional support are crucial for improving quality of life in PCOS patients. PCOS significantly affects women's physical and emotional health. Multidisciplinary management strategies and support systems are essential to enhance HRQOL and mitigate long-term health risks.

Keywords: *Polycystic Ovary Syndrome, Health-Related Quality of Life, Hormonal Imbalance, Menstrual Irregularities, Hyperandrogenism, Metabolic Complications.*

Presented as Oral Presentation

Targeted Cancer Therapy Via Copper-Complexed Polymeric Nanoparticles

Scan to View online

Presented by
Dr. S.Brito Raj
School of Pharmacy, Dhanalakshmi Srinivasan University, Trichy, Samayapuram, Tamil Nadu, India

Abstract

This study enhances the cancer-targeting efficiency of Sunitinib Malate, an oral multikinase inhibitor with limited bioavailability, by encapsulating it in copper complex-loaded polymeric nanoparticles using chitosan and PEG. In silico results demonstrated a strong copper-binding affinity (-7.5). The Sunitinib-Copper nanoparticles, produced via solvent evaporation, exhibited sizes of 9-300 nm, entrapment efficiencies above 83%, and *in-vitro* drug release exceeding 85%. MTT assays revealed superior efficacy for chitosan-based nanoparticles, reducing cell viability to 23.88% in A498 renal carcinoma cells. These copper-infused nanoparticles present a promising platform for precision-targeted delivery of Sunitinib Malate in cancer treatment.

Keywords: *Nanoparticles, Chitosan, PEG, Copper, Cancer.*

Presented as Oral Presentation

Innovative Approaches to Green Synthesis: Enhancing Pharmaceutical Development through Sustainable Chemistry

Scan to View online

Presented by
Ms. Shital Sampat Sangale
Assistant Professor, SSWPS, Chandrabhaga College of Pharmacy, Katphal Baramati, Pune-Dist, Maharashtra, India

Abstract

The pharmaceutical industry is increasingly recognizing the importance of sustainable practices in response to environmental challenges and regulatory pressures. This research explores innovative approaches to green synthesis, focusing on how sustainable chemistry can enhance pharmaceutical development. By emphasizing principles such as atom economy, waste reduction, and the use of renewable resources, we investigate novel synthetic methodologies that minimize ecological impact while maintaining drug efficacy. Key strategies include the application of biocatalysts, the development of solvent-free reactions, and the utilization of microwave-assisted synthesis to improve energy efficiency. Case studies highlight successful implementations of these approaches in real-world pharmaceutical contexts, demonstrating significant reductions in environmental footprints and operational costs. Furthermore, we discuss the integration of life cycle assessments in the early stages of drug development; ensuring sustainability is a foundational consideration. This research aims to provide a comprehensive framework for adopting green chemistry in pharmaceutical synthesis, ultimately contributing to a more sustainable future in drug development

Keywords: *Green synthesis, sustainable practices, biocatalysts, solvent-free reactions*

Presented as Oral Presentation

Bio Active Herbal Cream With Nanoparticles: " Assessing Its Potential For Skin Health And Inflammation Management"

Scan to View online

Presented by
Dr. K Swathi Priya
Srinivasa Rao College of Pharmacy,
Visakhapatnam, Andhra Pradesh, India

Abstract

The primary aim of this research was to evaluate the potential of active constitutes of a polyherbal extract containing Lagerstroemia speciosa (Banaba), Moringa oleifera seeds, and organic Mussaenda and to develop a natural polyherbal cream formulation enriched with titanium dioxide nanoparticles. This formulation seeks to optimize the yield of bioactive compounds that contribute to antioxidant, anti-inflammatory, and antimicrobial activities, ultimately creating a safe and effective topical product for managing oxidative stress, inflammation, and microbial infections. Phytochemical screening was performed to evaluate the presence of active constituents. The extraction process yielded concentrated extracts rich in bioactive compounds, which were subjected to various *in-vitro* assays to evaluate their antioxidant, anti-inflammatory, and antimicrobial properties. The incorporation of TiO_2 nanoparticles is anticipated to enhance the cream's protective capabilities against UV radiation while potentially improving the delivery of the herbal extracts.. Two methods were studied to estimate the anti-inflammatory power which showed a clear picture revealing the effects on inflammation. Future research is proposed to explore the underlying mechanisms of action, optimize formulation techniques, and assess the broader therapeutic applications of the cream.

Keywords *Lagerstroemia speciosa, Moringa oleifera seeds, Organic Mussaenda, Anti-inflammatory, Anti oxidant, Anti-microbial, Polyherbal, Formulation*

Presented as Oral Presentation

Development And *In-vitro* Assessment Of Zoledronic Acid Buccal Patches

Scan to View online

Presented by
Dr. Madhavi Latha Samala
Aditya College of Pharmacy, Aditya University, Surampalem, Andhra Pradesh, India

Abstract

Zoledronic acid (ZA) is a BCS class IV medication that serves as a bone resorption inhibitor with a low bioavailability of 5%, making it an excellent choice for buccal delivery. The purpose of this study is to develop and characterize oral mucoadhesive buccal patches containing zoledronic acid in order to improve medication permeability and bioavailability. Eight distinct formulations were created utilizing varying percentages of the polymers guar gum, xanthan gum, and HPMC. Polymer solutions in isopropyl alcohol were mixed with methanolic ZA solutions using a magnetic stirrer at 3000 rpm for 5 minutes in the presence of PEG as a plasticizer and Tween 80 as a surfactant until a semisolid consistency was achieved. The resulting mixture was cast in Teflon-coated glass molds. Physicochemical parameters include surface pH, swelling index, percent moisture absorption, folding endurance, patch thickness, *in-vitro* drug release studies and *in-vitro* mucoadhesion properties were evaluated. All the formulations exhibited acceptable physicochemical properties and the formulations prepared using xanthan gum 2% showed gradual and controlled *in-vitro* drug release pattern when compared to others. In conclusion, zoledronic acid can be delivered by buccal patch employing xanthan gum as controlled release and mucoadhesive polymer successfully.

Keywords: *Zoledronic acid, Buccal patch, Xanthan gum, Guar gum, HPMC, in-vitro drug release, in-vitro muco adhesion*

Presented as Oral Presentation

Chronotherapy And Personalized Care: A New Frontier In Precision Medicine

Scan to View online

Presented by
Dr. Rajeswari Aleti
Gokaraju Rangaraju College of Pharmacy,
Hyderabad, Telangana, India

Abstract

Chronotherapeutics in personalized medicine represents a transformative approach that integrates the body's circadian rhythms with individualized treatment strategies to optimize therapeutic outcomes. Biological processes such as hormone secretion, metabolism, and immune function follow circadian cycles, influencing the efficacy and toxicity of medications. Cardiovascular treatments, such as antihypertensives and statins, have demonstrated superior outcomes when administered based on the patient's circadian blood pressure and cholesterol patterns. The approach also shows promise in diabetes management, where insulin sensitivity and glucose metabolism fluctuate throughout the day. Personalized chronotherapeutics combines circadian biology with patient-specific data, including genetic markers, sleep patterns, and lifestyle factors, to tailor medication schedules. Emerging technologies, such as wearable devices and smart drug delivery systems, enable real-time monitoring and adjustment of treatment timing, further enhancing precision medicine. The integration of chronotherapeutics into personalized medicine not only maximizes drug efficacy but also minimizes adverse effects, improving overall patient outcomes. Ongoing research and technological innovation are essential for overcoming challenges related to individual circadian variability and practical implementation, paving the way for more effective, time-tailored therapeutic interventions.

Keywords: *chronotherapeutic, personalized medicine, circadian cycles, cancer*

Presented as Oral Presentation

Formulation Development And Evaluation Of Lipsticks Using Natural Edible Colorants

Scan to View online

Presented by
Mrs. Kamma Keerthi
Aditya College of Pharmacy, Aditya University, Surampalem, Andhra Pradesh, India

Abstract

Aim of the present research work is to formulate Lipsticks by using natural edible colorants from vegetable sources and evaluate them. In this study, 5 formulations are finalized after too many trials. Coloring matter was extracted from natural sources such as carrot, beetroot, turmeric and cocoa. Other natural ingredients such as beeswax, Carnauba wax, Cetyl alcohol, white soft paraffin, vanilla essence and vitamin E were used. Coconut oil, almond oil, and castor oil were tried in different combinations. Prepared Lipsticks were evaluated for Surface anomalies, Aging stability, Skin irritation test ,Color of the lipstick, Melting point, Hardness, Spread ability and Breaking point. From the results of evaluation test it was concluded that the formulation using castor oil and coconut oil blend with curcumin colorant (F4) was found to be the optimal formulation because of its color retention and stability likewise, even all the formulations also exhibited satisfactory results, but when compared with all the formulations F4 formulation exhibited good results.

Keywords: *Herbal lipstick, edible colorant, Natural ingredient, Formulation, Evaluation.*

Presented as Oral Presentation

Investigating The *In vivo* Anti-Amnesic Property Of Ethanolic Leaf Extract Of Ocimum Sanctum

Scan to View online

Presented by
Miss Kodi Gnaneswari
Aditya College of Pharmacy, Aditya University, Surampalem, Andhra Pradesh, India

Abstract

The current investigation aims to research the anti-amnesic activity of Ocimum sanctum leaf extract which possess Anti-amnesic activity against stress induced amnesia, learning and memory enhancing activity. Cook's pole climbing apparatus was used to determine this activity. It aids in determining both the animal's conditioned avoidance response (CAR) (climbing the pole after a buzzer with significant training, i.e., declarative training) and unconditioned response (climbing the pole after applying foot shock, i.e., procedural learning). Learning and Memory was evaluated by checking the transfer latency using Y-maze. The orally administered extract of Ocimum sanctum showed an increase in the number of CAR in less days and time due to the increase of acetylcholine content and thus improving the nootropic action in amnesia induced animal models. The current study provides scientific evidence in favour of the anti-amnesia activity of Ocimum sanctum leaf extract in treatment of amnesia.

Keywords: *Ocimum sanctum, Cook's pole climbing apparatus, Y-Maze, Conditioned Avoidance Response (CAR), Nootropic.*

Presented as Oral Presentation

Nipah Virus: A Zoonotic Threat To Global Health

Scan to View online

Presented by
Dr. Komala Aiswarya Kokku, J Bhargava Narendra
Aditya Pharmacy College, Aditya University, Surampalem, Andhra Pradesh, India

Abstract

A type of viral infection brought on by the Nipah virus is called a Nipah virus infection. It is an RNA virus belonging to the "Henipa Virus" genus. Some "fruit bats" are typically the carriers of the virus. One of the most deadly new zoonotic viruses and a possible danger to global health security is the Nipah Virus (NiV). NiV is a bat-borne pathogen (zoonotic virus) that can infect humans directly or through contaminated food, causing fatal encephalitis. A range of illnesses, from asymptomatic infections to fever, cough, headache, dyspnea, serious respiratory infections and deadly encephalitis, are brought on by the virus. Approximately 50 to 75 percent of infected individuals die, and they may go into coma within a day or two. First identified in Malaysia in 1998, the NiV was discovered in Siliguri, India, in 2001. It was then linked to a second outbreak in the Nadia District of West Bengal in 2007, and the current outbreak in Kerala claimed over 17 lives and afflicted several others. Brain inflammation and seizures after healing are examples of complications. In most cases, physical contact with an infected source is necessary for spread. The diagnosis is made based on the patient's symptoms and verified by laboratory tests such as RT-PCR, phylogenetic analysis, serologic analysis, and NiV sequencing. As of 2024, there is no licensed treatment or vaccination; therefore, management is limited to supportive care. Avoiding bats and sick pigs, as well as avoid drinking raw date palm sap, are preventive strategies.

Keywords: *Henipa Virus, Zoonotic Virus, Date Palm sap, Encephalitis.*

Presented as Oral Presentation

Validation Of UPLC-PDA Stability Indicating Method For Quantification Of Antiviral Drugs In Fixed Dose Combination

Scan to View online

Presented by
Dr. Divya Narla
Aditya College of Pharmacy, Aditya University, Surampalem, Andhra Pradesh, India

Abstract

The present research was focused on development of a validated stability indicating method for simultaneous quantification of Sofosbuvir, Velpatasvir and Voxilaprevir in bulk and tablet dosage form using UPLC. The separation of analytes was achieved on C18 BEH column (100×2.1mm, 1.7µm), with mobile phase consisting of phosphate buffer and acetonitrile in the ratio of 65:35v/v at a flow rate of 0.2ml/min. PDA detector was used to detect analytes at 265nm. The developed method was validated according to ICH guidelines. The method was linear over the concentration range of 100 - 600µg/ml for Sofosbuvir, 25 - 150µg/ml for Velpatasvir and Voxilaprevir. The retention times were found to be 0.908, 1.191 and 1.739mins for Sofosbuvir, Velpatasvir and Voxilaprevir respectively. The %RSD values for precision (Repeatability), accuracy and robustness were complying with limits. The LOD and LOQ were found to be 0.76 & 2.30 for Sofosbuvir, 0.61 & 1.85 for Velpatasvir and 0.49 & 1.47 for Voxilaprevir. Forced degradation was done on analytes under the conditions of acid, alkali, peroxide, thermal, UV and water. The results obtained were within limits and the analytes are detected without any interference from degradants. The method was successfully applied for the assay of VOSEVI tablets. Thus, the developed method allows the quantification of Sofosbuvir, Velpatasvir and Voxilaprevir in bulk and tablets even in the presence of degradants.

Keywords: *Sofosbuvir, Velpatasvir; Voxilaprevir, Stability indicating, UPLC, ICH.*

Presented as Oral Presentation

Emergent Roles Of Cuproptosis And Ferroptosis In Wilson Disease: Molecular Pathways And Clinical Consequences

Scan to View online

Presented by
Miss Bommeti Sara Aiswarya
Aditya Pharmacy College, Aditya University, Surampalem, Andhra Pradesh, India

Abstract

Wilson's disease, also known as hepatolenticular degeneration, is a congenital metabolic disorder rarely marked by elevated levels of copper in the body, directly in the liver and the brain, and it is life-threatening over time. Such an abundance of copper causes overproduction of reactive oxygen species (ROS) and cuproptosis that can kill the cells. Furthermore, elevated hepatic iron stores may lead to iron-mediated apoptosis by triggering phospholipid peroxidation in mitochondrial membranes and eventually causing ferroptosis, the accumulation of sulfur-rich organelle membranes. Inherited defective or absent ATP7B protein leads to impaired biliary excretion of copper and, thus, copper accumulation in the liver. Several clinical features are characteristic of Wilson disease (in parentheses); depression, psychosis, dysarthria, ataxia, writing difficulty, neuropsychiatric, dysphagia, renal tubular failure, Kayser–Fleischer corneal rings, cardiomyopathy and cardiac arrhythmias, rhabdomyolysis, Osteoporosis, osteomalacia, osteoarthritis, and arthralgia. Wilson's illness is diagnosed by the modified Leipzig Scoring System and the first therapy of choice is copper chelating agents like D-penicillamine. Prognosis is better when chelation treatment is prompt and liver transplantation is a treatment of last resort for advanced liver disease with intractable complications or sudden liver failure. Finally and most importantly, Wilson's disease is a multifactorial genetic disorder and as much a challenge at the levels of both its molecular and clinical diagnosis.

Keywords: *Wilson's disease, Cuproptosis, Ferroptosis, Kayser Fleischer corneal rings, Rhabdomyolysis, cardiomyopathy.*

Presented as Oral Presentation

Development & Evaluation of Taste Masked Formulation of Piroxicam

Scan to View online

Presented by
Mr. Hemantkumar Laxman Bhosale, Dr. Harshal Ashok Pawar
Mansarovar Global University, Billkisganj, Sehore, Bhopal, Madhya Pradesh, India

Abstract

Piroxicam, a potent nonsteroidal anti-inflammatory drug (NSAID), is widely used for the management of various inflammatory conditions. However, its bitter taste poses a significant challenge for patient compliance, particularly in pediatric and geriatric populations. In this study, we aimed to develop and evaluate a taste-masked formulation of piroxicam to enhance patient acceptability and adherence. Using a combination of taste-masking techniques including complexation, microencapsulation, and flavoring, we prepared several formulations of piroxicam. The optimized formulation demonstrated a significant reduction in bitterness while maintaining drug content and dissolution characteristics comparable to the unmasked drug. Sensory evaluation revealed improved palatability and acceptability of the taste-masked formulation compared to the unmasked drug. In conclusion, the developed taste-masked formulation of piroxicam presents a promising approach to overcome the taste aversion associated with this medication, potentially enhancing patient compliance and therapeutic outcomes, especially in vulnerable patient populations. Further studies including *in vivo* pharmacokinetic and pharmacodynamic evaluations are warranted to validate the clinical efficacy and safety of the formulated product

Keywords: *Taste masking, Piroxicam, Coating techniques, Oral dosage forms, Patient compliance*

Presented as Oral Presentation

Menstrual Hygiene And Health-Seeking Behaviour Among Medical Undergraduates: Addressing Knowledge And Practice Gaps

Scan to View online

Presented by
Miss Lalitha Maheswari Dandipati
Aditya Pharmacy College, Aditya University, Surampalem, Andhra Pradesh, India

Abstract

Menstrual health is a vital public health issue, especially in developing countries where cultural stigmas, limited access to sanitary products, and poor hygiene practices exist. Understanding the knowledge and practices of prospective healthcare professionals regarding menstrual hygiene is essential to improve menstrual health management (MHM) and health outcomes. This cross-sectional study involved 236 female medical students at Aditya Pharmacy College in Surampalem, Andhra Pradesh, from June to September 2024. Data were collected using a structured questionnaire via Google Forms, covering socio-demographic characteristics, menstrual hygiene practices, health-seeking behaviours, and the environmental impact of menstrual products. Statistical analysis was performed using SPSS version 20.0. Among the participants, 95.1% received menstruation education, and 92.1% discussed it with their mothers. While 95.7% were open to seeking medical help for menstrual issues, 39.4% missed college classes due to symptoms. Most (98.4%) used disposable pads, but only 10.5% were aware that menstrual cups can be reused for 5 to 6 years. The research highlights deficiencies in menstrual hygiene practices, particularly in hand washing and menstrual product disposal. Educational initiatives on menstrual hygiene, environmental impacts, and sustainable alternatives are essential. Improving access to healthcare and sanitary facilities enhances menstrual health management (MHM), resulting in better health outcomes and greater gender equality.

Keywords: *Menstrual hygiene, Undergraduate students, Dysmenorrhea, Health-seeking behaviour, Sustainable menstrual products*

Presented as Oral Presentation

Nano Emulsions - A Review

Scan to View online

Presented by
Miss Ummuri Bhavani
Vignan Institute of Pharmaceutical Technology, Visakhapatnam, Andhra Pradesh, India

Abstract

To overcome the difficulties associated with conventional drug delivery systems, an innovative and effective drug delivery has been created. Nanoemulsions, which are emulsions produced in nanoscales to enhance the administration of active medicinal components, are one of these drug delivery technologies.Any medicine can be made into a nanoemulsion systems, which has a greater surface area and better energy exchange and is a more effective way to distribute drugs. They made into thermodynamically stable systems by incorporating an emulsifying agent like a surfactant and a co-surfactant, that combine two immiscible liquids into a single phase. Nanoemulsions possess particle size in nanometers ranging from 20 to 200 nm. The properties of emulsion like Size and shape of the particle scattered in the continuous phase separates the emulsion from a nanoemulsion. Nano emulsions are used often in the sectors of medicine, food industry, cosmetics, agriculture, and other industries that require effective means or vehicles for protection.This review mainly deals with the concepts of Formulation involved in Nanoemulsion, preparation methods , characterization, evaluation procedure for prepared Nano emulsions, and their immense applications in various fields .

Keywords: *Nanoemulsions, Drug delivery, Types of emulsions, Applications.*

Presented as Oral Presentation

Crafting Nature'S Cleanser: Analyzing Cold-Pressed Herbal Soap Formulations With Natural Oils

Scan to View online

Presented by
Dr. D.Vasudha
Vignan Institute of Pharmaceutical Technology, Visakhapatnam, Andhra Pradesh, India

Abstract

This study explores the formulation of herbal soap using the cold process method, incorporating a blend of castor oil, coconut oil, palm oil, rose oil, tea tree oil, and a lye solution. The objective was to develop a soap with beneficial properties for skin care and to evaluate its effectiveness across various parameters. The formulated soap was subjected to a series of tests, including moisture content, pH stability, lathering capability, cleansing efficiency, foaming index, total fatty matter (TFM). The study aims to demonstrate the potential of these oils in enhancing skin health and treating skin conditions through regular use. The findings reveal the successful creation of a herbal soap with desirable qualities, showcasing its potential for both everyday use and therapeutic applications.

Keywords: *Herbal soap, pH lathering, dermatological infections, habitual use.*

Presented as Oral Presentation

Mesenchymal Stem Cells (Mscs) In Veterinary And Regenerative Medicine: A Review

Scan to View online

Presented by
Miss Sri Harshitha Manchala
Aditya Pharmacy College, Aditya University, Surampalem, Andhra Pradesh, India

Abstract

Recent advancements in stem cell research have opened new possibilities for treating diseases and conditions that currently lack effective treatments. Stem cells are unique in their ability to differentiate into various cell types, helping to replace damaged or aging cells in the body. Mesenchymal stem cells (MSCs), which can be easily extracted from adipose tissue and expanded in laboratory settings, have emerged as a promising tool for tissue repair and regeneration. MSCs have been widely used in animal studies and clinical trials, showing potential for cell-based therapies. This review aims to summarize the current knowledge about stem cells isolated from various animal models, including horses, pigs, goats, dogs, rabbits, cats, rats, and mice. Given the increasing focus on MSCs, this review will also discuss their use in veterinary medicine and regenerative therapies. MSCs have shown promise in treating conditions like heart failure, wound healing, and tooth regeneration.

Keywords: *Mesenchymal stem cells (MSCs), animal models, cell-based therapy, regenerative medicine*

Presented as Oral Presentation

Nanomedicine: Advancing Healthcare With Innovative Smart Pills

Scan to View online

Presented by
Mrs. B.Hema Kiranmayi
Aditya College of Pharmacy, Aditya University, Surampalem, Andhra Pradesh, India

Abstract

Nanomedicine is revolutionizing healthcare with its use of nanotechnology to develop sophisticated medical tools such as "smart pills". These nanoscale electronic devices, designed like pharmaceutical tablets, perform advanced tasks like drug delivery, sensing, and imaging. Innovations include dose-tracking pills and the "PillCam", equipped with a miniature video camera. The "Atmo Gas Capsule" analyses gut gases to detect abnormalities, diagnose gastrointestinal disorders and monitor-diet-related issues. MIT's "Smart Sensor Capsules" eliminate the need for stomach injections by unfolding and attaching to organs, tracking vital signs and releasing pre-loaded medications. Such advancements highlight nanotechnology's potential to enable real-time treatment and data collection, transforming science fiction into reality. Nano medicine not only promises to improve diagnosis and treatment but also offers personalized medicine options. Smart pills can target specific areas within the body, reducing side effects and increasing the efficacy of treatments. Additionally, these capsules can monitor patient compliance, ensuring that medications are taken as prescribed. The integration of such technology in healthcare lead to early detection of diseases ,better management of chronic conditions and overall improved patient outcomes. With continuous advancements, nanomedicine is set to play a crucial role in the future of healthcare making medical treatments more precise, less invasive and highly effective.

Keywords: *Smart Pill, Smart sensor Capsules, Precise, Dose-tracking.*

Presented as Oral Presentation

Formulation And Characterisation Of Herbal Nanoemulgel For Wound Healing Activity Using Punica Granatum And Jojoba Oil.

Scan to View online

Presented by
Mrs. Arumilli Swetha
Aditya College of Pharmacy, Aditya University, Surampalem, Andhra Pradesh, India

Abstract

The innovative technology made by converting nano-emulsion to nanoemulgel enhances stability and permits for both immediate and controlled release drug delivery. Nano-emulgel has also gained more attention because of its safety profile, convenience of use, lack of gastrointestinal breakdown or first-pass metabolism. Since ancient times, plant-based remedies have been used to heal a wide range of human illnesses. Therefore, the assessment of herbal plants' potential for creating novel dosage forms has led to the treatment of a number of illnesses. Therefore, the primary goal of this work was to formulate a topical emulgel using jojoba oil and Punica granatum herbal extracts because these extracts have the ability to treat wounds. Punica granatum peels were first extracted using the maceration method with ethanol solvent, and then the extract was purified using column chromatography with n-hexane solvent. Based on the solubility and emulsification ability, different nanoemulsion components (Oil, Surfactant and Cosurfactant) were selected. The nanoemulsion was prepared using high pressure homogenisation technique. Carbopol 934 was added to transform nanoemulsion into nanoemulgel. Then it was characterized and evaluated for pH, particle size, physical appearance, viscosity, spreadability, TEM, drug content, diffusion study, release kinetics, and stability studies. The physical characteristics, homogeneity, consistency, spreadability, viscosity, and pH value of all the prepared formulations were satisfactory.

Keywords: *Nanoemulgel, Punica granatum, jojoba wound Healing, extraction, Homogenization*

Presented as Oral Presentation

Elevated Creatine Kinase Due To Potential Drug Interaction With Ticagrelor And Atorvastatin

Scan to View online

Presented by
Miss Pushpa Satya Mahalakshmi Sanivarapu
Aditya Pharmacy College, Aditya University, Surampalem, Andhra Pradesh, India

Abstract

The two drugs commonly used in the management of acute coronary syndrome and percutaneous intervention are ticagrelor and atorvastatin. This case report is about a patient with the potential for having a drug interaction that would necessitate alternative care. Pharmacokinetic studies have shown a potential interaction between ticagrelor and atorvastatin but were not considered clinically significant. An interaction between atorvastatin and ticagrelor can cause severe rhabdomyolysis, which progresses to multiorgan failure. A 68-year-old female patient presented to the catheterization lab for cardiac catheterization after an abnormal stress test. He had placement of a drug-eluting stent and received initiation of ticagrelor. Three months later, his elevated creatine kinase (CK) was noted to likely represent a drug - drug interaction with atorvastatin. Ticagrelor was discontinued and he was transitioned successfully over to clopidogrel. CK returned to normal within weeks of this change. Atorvastatin and ticagrelor concomitantly administered, likely representing a drug-drug interaction. Although this interaction generally is not clinically significant, it should be part of the differential diagnosis for a patient presenting with signs and symptoms of adverse effects.

Keywords: *adverse drug reaction; atorvastatin; creatine kinase; drug interaction; ticagrelor.*

Presented as Oral Presentation

Hypovitaminosis D: A Hidden Complication In Chronic Kidney Disease

Scan to View online

Presented by
Miss Mounika Budati
Aditya Pharmacy College, Aditya University, Surampalem, Andhra Pradesh, India

Abstract

A growing public health concern, chronic kidney disease (CKD) is one of the strongest indicators of early cardiovascular disease. Maintaining healthy bones and muscles depends on vitamin D. The serum 25 hydroxyvitamin D (25OHD) levels are a sensitive indicator of the body's overall vitamin D reserves. There is growing evidence that hypovitaminosis D may be connected to the development of chronic kidney disease (CKD) and other cardiovascular problems. The decreased capacity to convert 25-(OH) vitamin D into the active form, 1,25 dihydroxy vitamin D, makes the remarkably high prevalence of severe vitamin D insufficiency in CKD patients even worse. It is clear that vitamin D's autocrine role is a significant modulator of several systems, including the immunological, renal, and cardiovascular systems, as recent research has deepened our understanding of both the classical and non-classical roles of the vitamin. The extremely high frequency of severe vitamin D insufficiency in CKD patients is exacerbated by the reduced ability to convert 25-(OH) vitamin D into the active form, 1,25 dihydroxy vitamin D. Recent studies have expanded our knowledge of the vitamin's classical and non-classical functions, making it evident that vitamin D's autocrine function is a major modulator of several systems, including the cardiovascular, renal, and immune systems.

Keywords: *Vitamin D, Chronic Kidney Disease, Cardiovascular, hypovitaminosis D,25 hydroxyvitamin D (25OHD)*

Presented as Oral Presentation

Drug-Drug Cocrystals: Advancing Combination Treatments And Improving Patient Outcomes

Scan to View online

Presented by
Dr. Monika Nijhawan
Gokaraju Rangaraju College of Pharmacy,
Hyderabad, Telangana, India

Abstract

A drug-drug cocrystal (DDC) is a crystalline structure formed by two or more active pharmaceutical ingredients (APIs) in a fixed stoichiometric ratio, held together by non-covalent interactions such as hydrogen bonds, or van der Waals forces. This novel approach aims to optimize the physicochemical properties of both drugs simultaneously, enhancing their solubility, stability, and bioavailability. Drug-drug cocrystals hold significant promise in improving the effectiveness of combination therapies, reducing the pill burden for patients, and simplifying drug regimens. Drug-drug cocrystals can also offer synergistic therapeutic effects by combining drugs with complementary mechanisms of action, thereby enhancing efficacy while minimizing side effects. This is particularly beneficial in chronic diseases such as HIV, tuberculosis, and cancer. However, challenges remain in the design and regulatory approval of drug-drug cocrystals, as careful testing is required to ensure the safety, stability, and compatibility of the combined drugs. Despite these challenges, drug-drug cocrystals represent a promising strategy for optimizing combination therapies, improving patient adherence, and enhancing drug performance, paving the way for the next generation of pharmaceutical formulations. As research advances, drug-drug cocrystals could revolutionize the treatment of complex diseases and improve therapeutic outcomes.

Keywords: *Cocrystals, bioavailability, stability, solubility, drug*

Presented as Oral Presentation

Prednisolone Tablet Formulation and Assessment for Colon-Targeted Drug Delivery System

Scan to View online

Presented by
Dr. Ravi Dnyandeo Hole
Associate Professor, Institute of Pharmaceutical Science and Research (For Girls), Bhigwan, Dist-Pune, Maharashtra, India

Abstract

Preparing prednisolone pH-dependent release tablets and assessing their benefits as a colon-targeted medication delivery system were the goals of this study. Prednisolone, which is unstable in the stomach environment and insoluble in water, was combined to create pH-dependent tablets coated in Eudragit L100 and Eudragit S100, two methacrylic acid copolymers. Prednisolone's *in-vitro* release rate from coated tablets was examined in relation to the coating levels, polymer combination ratios, and core tablet compositions. Less than 10% of the medication was released in 0.1 N HCl within two hours, while around 90% of the drug was released in the pH 7.2 phosphate buffer within six hours, according to the data. For the treatment of colonic illness and oral drug administration that is unstable or prone to enzymatic degradation in the upper gastrointestinal tract, colon drug delivery is beneficial. In this investigation, coated tablets that dissolve readily in colonic pH were found to be resistant to gastric and small intestine pH circumstances. The current study's findings have shown that the pH-dependent tablet system is a viable means of reducing prednisolone's rapid hydrolysis in the stomach environment and enhancing the drug's oral bioavailability for the treatment of ulcerative colitis

Keywords: *Enteric coating, colon focused drug delivery, in-vitro dissolution, PH-dependent delivery mechanism, prednisolone*

Presented as Oral Presentation

Forumulation And Evaluation Of Antitussive Lozenges Using Aqueous Bark Extract Of Syzygium Cumini

Scan to View online

Presented by

Dr. Gana Manjusha Kondepudi
Vignan Institute of Pharmaceutical Technology, Visakhapatnam, Andhra Pradesh, India

Abstract

Syzygium cumini (S. cumini) (L.) Skeels (jambolan) is one of the widely used medicinal plants in the treatment of various diseases in particular diabetes. The genus Syzygium is one of the genera of the myrtle family Myrtaceae which is native to the tropics, particularly to tropical America and Australia. The aim of this research is to extract Syzygium cumini bark using maceration, pressurized liquid extraction and Ultrasound Assissted Extraction and to formulate and evaluate antitussive lozenges using the aqueous extract. 26.92g yield was obtained by pressurized liquid extraction which was the highest when compared to the yield obtained from the other two extractions. Thus pressurized liquid extraction was found to be the best technique out of the three extraction techniques used. The extracts obtained from maceration, pressurized liquid extraction and ultrasonication was subjected to preliminary phytochemical analysis, which confirmed the presence of saponins, flavanoids, alkaloids and tannins in all the three extracts. Hard lozenges and soft lozenges were prepared by incorporating the bark extract and were evaluated for physical appearance, friability and weight variation. The friability and weight variation of the hard and soft lozenges were within the limit.

Keywords: *Herbal lozenges, Syzygium cumini, anti tussive, pressurized liquid extraction, Ultra sound assissted extraction,*

Presented as Oral Presentation

Breast Cancer: A Multifaceted Disease

Scan to View online

Presented by
Miss Rangala Mohini
Vignan Institute of Pharmaceutical Technology, Visakhapatnam, Andhra Pradesh, India

Abstract

Carcinoma of the breast is a condition when the breast's cells proliferate uncontrollably. Breast cancer comes in various forms. Which breast cells develop into cancer determines the type of breast cancer. The majority of cases of breast cancer occur in the lobules or ducts. The most prevalent type of cancer in women 70% to 80% of instances of breast cancer worldwide when detected in the early stages and does not spread to other parts of the body. Advanced breast carcinoma with distant organ lesions is considered incurable with present therapies. Numerous biological traits of breast cancer include the activation of hormone receptors. (Progesterone and oestrogen receptors), BRCA mutations, and/or receptor 2 for human epidermal growth hormone (HER2, encoded by ERBB2). Molecular subtype influences the different treatment approaches. Systemic therapy and loco regional (surgery and radiation therapy) techniques are part of the multidisciplinary management of breast cancer. Exemplary systemic drugs include chemotherapy, anti-HERZ therapy, bone-stabilizing medications, poly (ADP-ribose) polymerase inhibitors among people with BRCA mutations, and, more recently, immunotherapy. Future methods of curing breast cancer must aim to achieve individualized treatment strategies, treatment de-escalation and escalation based on cancer biology, and early therapy response.

Keywords: *Breast cancer, Biological traits, mutations,therapies*

Presented as Oral Presentation

Applications Of Ethosomal Drug Delivery Systems As Novel Vesicular Carriers For Improved Transdermal Permeation

Scan to View online

Presented by
Mr. Prakash Nathaniel Kumar Sarella
Aditya College of Pharmacy, Aditya University, Surampalem, Andhra Pradesh, India

Abstract

Ethosomes have emerged as an innovative vesicular drug delivery system, offering significant advantages in transdermal drug administration. These malleable vesicles, composed of phospholipids, ethanol, and water, demonstrate superior skin penetration capabilities compared to conventional liposomes. The unique composition of ethosomes, particularly their high ethanol content (20-45%), enables efficient drug entrapment and enhanced skin permeation through multiple mechanisms. The presence of ethanol fluidizes both the ethosomal lipid bilayers and intercellular lipids in the stratum corneum, facilitating deeper penetration of drug molecules. Various preparation techniques, including the cold method, hot method, and thin-film hydration method, have been developed to optimize ethosomal formulations. Ethosomes have shown particular promise in delivering anti-inflammatory drugs, antifungal agents, antibiotics, and anticancer drugs through the transdermal route. The system's ability to enhance drug permeation while maintaining stability makes it especially suitable for compounds with poor skin penetration profiles or those requiring sustained release. Additionally, ethosomes exhibit minimal toxicity and skin irritation, supporting their safety profile for pharmaceutical applications. Despite these advantages, challenges remain in large-scale manufacturing and stability optimization.

Keywords: *Ethosomes, Transdermal delivery, Vesicular carriers, Skin penetration, Drug encapsulation*

Presented as Oral Presentation

Preliminary Phyochemical Screening And Evaluation Of Anti-Inflammatory, Analgeic And Anti-Pyretic Properties Of Eugenia Jambolana Seeds Extract In Albino Rats.

Scan to View online

Presented by
Mrs. S.Thirumala Devi
Aditya College of Pharmacy, Aditya University, Surampalem, Andhra Pradesh, India

Abstract

Eugenia jambolana commonly known as Black plum has wide range of medical uses. In order to provide a scientific rationale for the plants we looked into the anti-inflammatory, analgesic and anti-pyretic therapeutic properties of the seed extract. The extract exhibited the presence of alkaloids, tri-terpeniods, tannins, carbohydrates and proteins, as per the phytochemical study performed indicating a key role in the reduction of inflammation, nociception. The standard Acetic Acid Induced Writing Response Test was used to generate the anti-nociceptive activity, while the Carrageenan-induced paw oedema test was used to evaluate the anti-inflammatory and the Brewer's yeast suspension was used to induce the anti-pyretic activity in the mice. When compared to control and standard drug, the ethanolic seed extract of species showed the most therapeutic activity against inflammation, analgesia and pyrexia. We concluded that the ethanolic seed extracts of Eugenia jambolana have therapeutic efficacy for anti-inflammatory, analgesic and anti-pyretic activities in albino rats both *In vivo* and *In vivo* after analyzing the findings.

Keywords: *Eugenia jambolana, Anti-inflammatory, Analgesic, Anti-pyretic, Brewer's yeast*

Presented as Oral Presentation

Antibacterial Potentiation And Wound Healing Competence Through Bio-Mediated Zno Nanoparticle By Leaf Extract

Scan to View online

Presented by
Dr. Koppala Rvs Chaitanya
Sarojini Naidu Vanitha Pharmacy Maha Vidyalaya, Secunderabad, Telangana, India

Abstract

Zinc Oxide (ZnO) is presently utilized in nano-cosmeceuticals and nano-pharmaceuticals applied topically due to their versatile effectiveness, regardless of the method of synthesis. Hence, the aim of the current research is to produce ZnO nanoparticles (NPs) using a more environmentally friendly method employing Barleria cristata (BC) leaf extract in varying concentrations (2.5g, 5.0g, 7.0g, and 10.0g) and to assess their ability to enhance antibiotic effectiveness and combat cancer. The innovative synthesis of ZnO NPs was conducted without the use of any chemicals or high-temperature processing, under continuous stirring and refluxion in an oxygen-rich environment. BC is known for its medicinal phytochemicals, and thus, the incorporation of secondary metabolites onto ZnO NPs during synthesis as reducing, stabilizing, and capping agents may provide additional biomedical benefits. The synthesized BCZnO NPs were characterized by a characteristic peak at 375 nm in the absorbance spectra, as well as SEM and particle size analysis revealing particles ranging from 20 to 50 nm in size, possessing a hexagonal crystalline structure, and containing various phytochemicals and functional groups. Additionally, the antibacterial activity and antibiotic-potentiating capability of BC-ZnO NPs were investigated through combinational assays. Moreover, the wound healing potential of BC-ZnO NPs was evaluated using excision and incision wound models.

Keywords: *barleria cristata, SEM, Zinc Oxide, nanoparticles, wound healing*

Presented as Oral Presentation

Comparision Of Qualitative And Quantitative Analysis And *In vivo* Anti-Diabetic Activity Of Poly Herbal Mixtures Of Some Selected Herbs

Scan to View online

Presented by
Mrs. V. Jhansi Lakshmi
Gitam school of Pharmacy,
Vishakapatnam, Andhra Pradesh, India

Abstract

This study aimed to compare the results of the phytochemical screening of three medicinal plants (Ocimum sanctum, Aegelmarmelos, Syzygiumcumini) using ethanol: water in an aqueous hydroalcoholic solution [70:30] solvent. These plants were selected because they are widely distributed and accessible. Ocimum sanctum has historical relevance as a religious, cultural, and healing concept. Aegelmarmelos is used for a variety of therapeutic purposes, such as treating asthma, anemia, bone fractures, wound healing, joint swelling, high blood pressure, etc. These plants have been found to have many common phytochemicals such as flavonoids, tannins, saponins, alkaloids, etc. The results of the current study's thin layer chromatographic examination of ethanolic, hydroalcoholic, and aqueous polyherbal mixtures, which included flavonoids and glycosides, showed that Rf was less than 1, according to the analysis. The inhibitory effect brought on polyherbal mixtures was contrasted with Acarbose as a control for oral alpha-glucosidase and alpha-amylase inhibitors for the management of T2D. A complex oligosaccharide called Acarbose slows and lessens intestinal sugar absorption. Ethanolic, hydroalcoholic, and aqueous polyherbal mixtures' relative percentage of inhibition compared to Acarbose. Among the three Poly herbal hydroalcoholic mixtures, IC50 46.2, Polyherbal ethanolic mixture IC50 51.9, Polyherbal aqueous mixtures, IC50 58.9.

Keywords: *Polyherbal mixtures, Diabetes mellitus, Alpha-amylase, Medicinal herbs, Acarbose*

Presented as Oral Presentation

Navigating The Shadows Of Eating Disorders: An In-Depth Exploration Of Anorexia And Bulimia Nervosa

Scan to View online

Presented by
Dr. G Urmila
Vignan Institute of Pharmaceutical Technology, Visakhapatnam, Andhra Pradesh, India

Abstract

Anorexia nervosa and Bulimia nervosa are two of the most common and serious eating disorders that affect individuals, predominantly adolescents and young adults. These disorders are characterized by distinct patterns of disorder eating behaviours and preoccupation having profound impact on an individual's physical and mental well-being, and they often co-exist with other mental health conditions. Timely intervention and comprehensive treatment are essential to address these complex and potentially life-threatening conditions. The incidence of anorexia nervosa is increasing in younger people [aged <15years]. During their lifetime, up to 4% of females and up to 0.3% of males suffer from anorexia nervosa and up to 3% of females and more than 1% of males from bulimia nervosa. Both disorders involve distorted body images and unhealthy eating behaviours. Early intervention comprehensive treatment can lead to improved outcomes and a higher quality of live for those struggling with anorexia and bulimia nervosa.

Keywords: *Anorexia nervosa, Bulimia nervosa, young adults, nutritional rehabilitation*

Presented as Oral Presentation

Development And Evaluation Of Bilayer Transdermal Patches Of Canagliflozin Using Hpmc Grades For Sustained Drug Delivery

Scan to View online

Presented by
Dr. Venna R Surya Anusha
Gokaraju Rangaraju College of Pharmacy,
Hyderabad, Telangana, India

Abstract

This study investigates the formulation and evaluation of transdermal patches for the controlled delivery of canagliflozin, an SGLT2 inhibitor used in diabetes management, employing different grades of hydroxypropyl methylcellulose (HPMC) via a bilayer technique. Transdermal systems offer advantages such as improved bioavailability, reduced dosing frequency, and avoidance of first-pass metabolism, addressing the limitations of oral drug administration. Patches were prepared by solvent casting, with the drug-loaded layer formulated using HPMC K4M and HPMC E15, and a non-drug-containing backing layer. The results indicated that HPMC K4M-based patches exhibited higher mechanical strength and moisture retention, while HPMC E15-based patches showed enhanced flexibility. Drug release studies revealed a sustained release profile over 24 hours, with the HPMC E15 formulation releasing 85% of the drug, compared to 72% for HPMC K4M. Permeation studies demonstrated efficient transdermal delivery, with optimized formulations achieving a steady permeation rate, ensuring prolonged systemic absorption. In conclusion, the transdermal patches developed using the bilayer technique and HPMC grades provided a controlled and sustained release of canagliflozin, making them a promising alternative to oral therapy for diabetes management.

Keywords: *Hydroxypropyl methylcellulose; Transdermal patch; canagliflozin; Bilayer patches; Sustained Drug Delivery;*

Presented as Oral Presentation

Artificial Intelligence Tools In Pharmacovigilance

Scan to View online

Presented by
Dr. Priyadarshini
Vignan Institute of Pharmaceutical Technology, Visakhapatnam, Andhra Pradesh, India

Abstract

Artificial intelligence (AI) tools in pharmacovigilance has emerged as a transformative approach to enhancing drug safety monitoring. As adverse drug reactions (ADRs) pose significant public health risks, AI-driven methodologies facilitate the rapid identification, assessment, and management of these events. Techniques such as natural language processing (NLP) enable the extraction of relevant information from unstructured data sources, including electronic health records and social media. Machine learning algorithms further enhance signal detection by analyzing large datasets to identify patterns indicative of potential safety issues. Additionally, AI can automate routine tasks, allowing pharmacovigilance professionals to focus on more complex analyses and decision-making processes. This abstract highlights the potential benefits and challenges associated with integrating AI into pharmacovigilance, emphasizing the need for robust regulatory frameworks to ensure data integrity and patient safety. Continued research and collaboration among stakeholders are essential to fully realize the advantages of AI in this critical field.

Keywords: *Artificial Intelligence , Drug safety, Adverse drug reactions , Pharmacovigilance*

Presented as Oral Presentation

Comparative Study Of Myocardial Infarction In Smoker And Non Smoker Patients

Scan to View online

Presented by
Miss Adabala Gaana Lakshmi
Aditya College of Pharmacy, Aditya University, Surampalem, Andhra Pradesh, India

Abstract

Myocardial infarction (MI), commonly known as a heart attack, occurs when blood flow through the coronary arteries is significantly reduced, leading to tissue damage and ischemia. This reduction often results from the formation of an atherosclerotic plaque, which can trigger the development of a thrombus and block the artery. Cigarette smoking exacerbates this risk by increasing heart rate and blood pressure while constricting coronary arteries and impairing blood flow. Research indicates that smokers are more likely to experience MI and present with symptoms such as chest pain, shortness of breath, and excessive sweating. The majority of MI cases among smokers involve males, who face a significantly higher risk compared to non-smokers. In terms of treatment, antiplatelet and anticoagulant medications were most frequently prescribed, followed by fibrinolytics and thrombolytics. Additional medications included anti-anginal drugs, narcotics, beta-blockers, statins, ACE inhibitors, and calcium channel blockers the latter being the most common choice among antihypertensives. The study sought to determine the relation between smoking and nonsmoking in myocardial infraction and also found that non-smokers tend to experience milder symptoms and shorter recovery periods. They respond more effectively to treatment, while smokers typically require higher medication doses. Smokers in the study were predominantly male, aged between 31 and 60 years.

Keywords: *myocardial infraction, atherosclerosis, smoking, ischemia*

Presented as Oral Presentation

Dual Viral Assault: A Case Of Acute Liver Failure From Dengue And Hepatitis A Coinfection

Scan to View online

Presented by
Dr. Nandini Palivela
Aditya College of Pharmacy, Aditya University, Surampalem, Andhra Pradesh, India

Abstract

Acute liver failure (ALF) is a rare and diverse condition that affects people without a history of liver disease. It is characterized by a significant impairment of liver function. This case study describes a unique instance of ALF caused by co-infection with the dengue virus and hepatitis A virus (HAV), which is also associated with dengue hemorrhagic fever. The 24-year-old male patient presented with symptoms that included fever, nausea, vomiting, abdominal pain, and widespread body aches. Subsequently, the patient developed jaundice, hepatic encephalopathy, acute cholecystitis, and acute pancreatitis. Tests in the lab verified the presence of dengue and HAV markers as well as lower hemoglobin and platelet counts. Nonetheless, the patient's condition progressively improved under a conservative management-focused treatment plan, which ultimately resulted in discharge. In order to achieve the best possible outcomes for the patient, this case highlights the possibility that coinfection with dengue and HAV could cause ALF. It also highlights the importance of early diagnosis and prompt intervention.

Keywords: *Acute liver failure, Dengue virus, Hepatitis A virus, coinfection, Intensive care*

Presented as Oral Presentation

In vivo Anti-Anemic Activity Of Ethanolic Root And Leaf Extracts Of Taraxacum Officinale In Phenylhydrazine Induced Anemic Rats

Scan to View online

Presented by
Mrs. S Thirumala Devi
Aditya College of Pharmacy, Aditya University, Surampalem, Andhra Pradesh, India

Abstract

Dandelion (Taraxacum officinale) is a highly beneficial plant for improving blood health and addressing anemia. Both the root and leaves of the dandelion have therapeutic properties, particularly due to their high iron content and ability to support liver function. The present work was carried out to evaluate the *in vivo* Anti-anaemic activity of Taraxacum officinale leaf and root extracts in Phenylhydrazine induced anaemic rats. The ethanolic extract at a high and low dose of 200 and 400 mg/kg showed an increased the iron content by showing a remarkable elavation in the production of hemoglobin, red blood cells and percentage of hematocrit which was analyzed by the hematology analyzer in comparision to the Phenylhydrazine treated animals group and the results are comparable with that of standard vitamin B12 complex. Thus, the present study reveals that the ethanolic leaf and root extract of Taraxacum officinale is suitable for administration for treating anemia condition.

Keywords: *Taraxacum officinale, Phenylhydrazine, Anaemia, Hematology analyzer, Hemoglobin, Hematocrit.*

Presented as Oral Presentation

The Impact Of Age On Lung Function In Chronic Obstructive Pulmonary Disease (Copd) Patients

Scan to View online

Presented by
Miss A.B.S.D Padma Sri
Aditya College of Pharmacy, Aditya University, Surampalem, Andhra Pradesh, India

Abstract

COPD is a prevalent respiratory condition affecting millions, particularly those aged 44-65. To investigate the effect of age on lung function in COPD patients compared to healthy individuals. A six-month study (Oct 2023-Mar 2024) at GSL General Hospital and Medical College, Rajahmundry, included 52 participants (26 COPD patients, 26 healthy individuals) aged 20-80. Spirometry and St. George's Respiratory Questionnaire (SGRQ) assessed lung function and quality of life. COPD patients showed significant declines in lung function, quality of life, and increased symptoms with advancing age. Shortness of breath affected 54% of patients. Chi-square tests and t-tests revealed significant associations between age and lung function parameters ($p < 0.001$). Age significantly impacts lung function in COPD patients, emphasizing the need for early interventions, effective management strategies, and tailored therapeutic approaches for the elderly population.

Keywords: COPD, lung function, aging, quality of life, SGRQ, spirometry.

Presented as Oral Presentation

Anxiolytic Effect Of Ethanolic Whole Plant Extract Of Bacopa Monnieri Using Mice Model

Scan to View online

Presented by
Miss Kodi Gnaneswari
Aditya College of Pharmacy, Aditya University, Surampalem, Andhra Pradesh, India

Abstract

Bacopa monnieri, also known as Brahmi, is a well-known herb in traditional Ayurvedic medicine, particularly for its cognitive and calming effects. It has gained recognition for its potential anti-anxiety properties, supported by modern research. The anxiolytic activity is evaluated using elevated plus maze and hole board test using Albino mice. The ethanolic whole plant extract of Bacopa monnieri at a dose of 75 and 150 mg/kg has shown more time spent and increased number of entries in the open arm using elevated plus maze in comparison to that of control group. In addition to this a significant reduction in latency to first nose poking was observed in the extract of 75 and 150 mg/kg with augmentation in head dipping behavior of control group. The results are compared with that of standard drug Diazepam 2mg/kg where the extract has shown promising results of anti-anxiety effects, primarily through its adaptogenic properties which it helps in coping with stress and promotes mental resilience and also the increases' ability to balance the neurotransmitters and shows the cognitive benefits of Bacopa monnieri.

Keywords: *Bacopa monnieri, Elevated plus maze, Hole board test, Adaptogenic, Anxiety, Nose poking.*

Presented as Oral Presentation

Advances In Lipid Nanocarriers: Targeted Therapeutic Strategies For Breast Cancer Treatment

Scan to View online

Presented by
Mr. Gummadi Ramakrishna
Aditya Pharmacy College, Aditya University, Surampalem, Andhra Pradesh, India

Abstract

Breast cancer is one of the most widespread cancers worldwide, and many of the current treatments are challenged by issues like drug resistance, unwanted side effects, and limited efficacy .Lipid-based nanocarriers (have gained attention as a promising solution for delivering chemotherapy drugs and biological molecules with improved targeting and precision. This review examines the role of lipid nano carriers, such as liposomes, solid lipid nanoparticles (SLNs), and nanostructured lipid carriers (NLCs), in advancing breast cancer treatment. These carriers, which encapsulate drugs with in lipid structures, enhance drug solubility, stability, and bioavailability while reducing harmful side effects. In addition, by modifying the surface of these nanocarriers, they can actively target cancer-specific receptors such as HER2, EGFR, and folate receptors, leading to more precise and effective treatment outcomes. The review outlines the recent progress in lipid nanocarrier technology, particularly in their ability to overcome biological barriers and improve treatment success, with a focus on the aggressive and hard-to –treat triple negative breast cancer (TNBC). It is also considers future developments in this area. Including combination therapies and systems responsive to specific stimuli, highlighting their potential in advancing personalized treatments for breast cancer

Keywords: *Breast cancer, Lipid nanocarriers, Targeted therapy, TNBC, Stimuli responsive system.*

Presented as Oral Presentation

Hydrogel Scaffolds: The Next Frontier In Tissue Regeneration

Scan to View online

Presented by
Mrs. B.Hema Kiranmayi
Aditya College of Pharmacy, Aditya University, Surampalem, Andhra Pradesh, India

Abstract

Hydrogel scaffolds are emerging as a pivotal tool in tissue engineering and regenerative medicine. These three-dimensional, water-swollen polymer networks mimic the extracellular matrix, providing a conducive environment for cell proliferation, differentiation, and tissue regeneration. Their highly porous structure facilitates nutrient and waste exchange, crucial for maintaining cell viability and function Hydrogel. One of the significant advantages of hydrogel scaffolds is their injectability, enabling minimally invasive delivery to target sites. Additionally, they can be loaded with bioactive molecules, such as growth factors and drugs, to enhance tissue repair processes. Advanced fabrication techniques, including 3D printing and electrospinning allow precise control over scaffold architecture, further improving their functionality. Recent studies have demonstrated the potential of hydrogel scaffolds in various applications, including cartilage repair, wound healing, and the regeneration of neural and cardiac tissues. Despite their promising attributes challenges remain such as long -term stability, controlling degradation rates and achieving uniform cell distribution within the scaffold. Future research aims to address these issues, potentially incorporating smart materials that respond to environmental stimuli, further broadening the clinical applicability of hydrogel scaffolds.

Keywords: *Hydrogel Scaffolds, Tissue regeneration, Biodegradability, 3D printing, Bioactive molecules.*

Presented as Oral Presentation

Formulation And Evaluation Of Acetazolamide Nanoparticulate Ocular In Situ Gel

Scan to View online

Presented by
Dr. J. Anu Pravallika
Aditya College of Pharmacy, Aditya University, Surampalem, Andhra Pradesh, India

Abstract

The aim of the present study is to formulate and evaluate ocular in situ gel-forming of acetazolamide nanosuspension using nanoprecipitation technique. Acetazolamide a carbonic anhydrase inhibitor is used to treat glaucoma, a neurodegenerative disorder peculiarized by increase in intraocular pressure. Carbopol 934 is the pH sensitive gelling agent used, which enhanced the ocular bioavailability. Eudragit RS 100 and Eudragit RL100 acts as release retardants were used in different concentrations. The FTIR studies showed that there are no interactions between drug and the polymers. The prepared in situ gel formulations were evaluated for clarity, pH, gelling capacity, SEM analysis, Zeta potential, *in-vitro* diffusion studies, drug entrapment efficiency and antimicrobial studies. The developed formulations were clear, transparent, and colorless moreover pH was found to be within the range of 7.1 to 7.4 which is acceptable. Among all, the formulation (F7) prepared with Eudragit RL100 shows best results and exhibits sustained drug release over a period of 6 hours with increasing residence time of the drug. These formulations may give a viable alternative to the conventional eye drops by virtue of its ability to sustain drug release for good stability and biocompatibility characteristics.

Keywords: *Acetazolamide, in situ gel, nanosuspensions, Eudragit, carbopol 934, nanoprecipitation technique*

Presented as Oral Presentation

Rare Case Report: Uncommon Manifestation Of Hypersplenism In Adult Patients With Sickle Cell Disease

Scan to View online

Presented by
Miss Mercy Pinipe
Aditya Pharmacy College, Aditya University, Surampalem, Andhra Pradesh, India

Abstract

Hypersplenism refers to the accelerated and premature breakdown of blood cells, characterized by a triad that includes splenomegaly, cytopenias, and increased bone marrow activity as a compensatory response. Sickle cell disease encompasses various genotypes, among which hemoglobin sickle C disease (HbSC) is characterized by the presence of both hemoglobin S and hemoglobin C. A 41-year-old female patient with a history of splenomegaly presented to the general surgery clinic due to abdominal pain. An acute splenic sequestration crisis may arise from hypersplenism, representing a potentially life-threatening complication associated with sickle hemoglobinemia. The ongoing cycle of sickle cell entrapment and stasis leads to multiple splenic infarctions, forming scar tissue within the splenic parenchyma. This process diminishes both the size and functionality of the spleen, ultimately culminating in auto-splenectomy. Our patient's spleen was measured at 21.1 cm, exceeding the typical size of an adult spleen. In this instance, the use of preoperative splenic artery embolization likely played a significant role in reducing intraoperative blood loss during the splenectomy, thereby lessening the requirement for transfusions during the perioperative period.

Keywords: *Hypersplenism, sickle cell disease, Slenomegaly, Splenic artery embolization, Splenectomy .*

Presented as Oral Presentation

Incidence And Risk Factors Of Tramadol-Induced Hypoglycemia: An Observational Study

Scan to View online

Presented by
Mr. Londa Eswar Naga Sai Datta Yadav
Aditya College of Pharmacy, Aditya University, Surampalem, Andhra Pradesh, India

Abstract

Tramadol is an analgesic commonly used for pain management, but it has been associated with rare adverse effects, including hypoglycemia. This observational study aims to assess the incidence of tramadol-induced hypoglycemia among patients and identify potential risk factors. A retrospective review was conducted at a tertiary care hospital, examining the medical records of patients prescribed tramadol over a one-year period. Patients were included if they experienced hypoglycemia (defined as blood glucose < 70 mg/dL) during tramadol treatment. Data on demographics, comorbidities, concurrent medications, and tramadol dosage were analyzed. Among 350 patients receiving tramadol, 15 (4.3%) experienced hypoglycemia. The average age of affected patients was 62 years, with a higher prevalence in those with diabetes (73.3%). Concomitant use of other medications affecting glucose metabolism, such as sulfonylureas, was noted in 60% of cases. Hypoglycemia episodes occurred more frequently with higher tramadol doses (>300 mg/day). The findings suggest that tramadol can induce hypoglycemia, particularly in older adults and those with diabetes or on other glucose-lowering medications. Awareness of this potential side effect is essential for healthcare providers when prescribing tramadol. Tramadol-induced hypoglycemia is a significant concern in certain patient populations. Monitoring blood glucose levels in high-risk patients is recommended to prevent adverse events.

Keywords: *Tramadol, Hypoglycemia, Observational study, Pain management, Diabetes, Risk factors, Concomitant medications,*

Presented as Oral Presentation

Studies On Fast Dissolving Tablets Of Promethazine Hydrochloride Formulated By Sublimation Technique

Scan to View online

Presented by
Dr. G Chandra Sekhara Rao
Vignan Institute of Pharmaceutical Technology, Visakhapatnam, Andhra Pradesh, India

Abstract

Fast dissolving drug delivery systems have gained patient acceptability and popularity in recent times. Antihistamine or anti emetic drugs like promethazine HCl have the oral problems like difficulty in swallowing, less oral bioavailability, first pass metabolism in conventional tablet dosage forms. To overcome such problems the antiemetic drugs can be formulated in the form of fast dissolving tablets where the drug is rapidly disintegrated in mouth within fraction of seconds and improves the onset of action and oral drug bioavailability. The purpose of this work was to develop oral fast dissolving tablets of promethazine HCl. Promethazine is an antiemetic drug especially used for motion sickness. Here an attempt has been made to prepare fast dissolving tablets by direct compression method using camphor as subliming agent in two concentrations of 8% and 10%. Crosspovidone and Pregelatinised starch are used as superdisintiegrants in different ratios (5%, 7.5%, and 10%). All prepared formulations were evaluated for weight variation, hardness, friability, drug content, disintegration time, wetting time, and in –vitro dissolution. The results obtained were within the limits. F7 was found to be the best formulation from the present study. The drug release followed first order kinetics. Sublimation technique was found to be suitable in the formulation of promethazine hydrochloride fast dissolving tablets.

Keywords: *Direct compression, Dissolution studies, fast dissolving tablets, Promethazine Hydrochloride, Superdisintegrants.*

Presented as Oral Presentation

Novel Pyrrolidine Schiff Bases synthesis Using Tamarind Extract as Eco-friendly Catalyst: Anti-oxidant activity & Molecular Docking Studies

Scan to View online

Presented by

Dr. Srikanth Kumar Karumanchi, Dr. Vishal Bharat Babar*

Professor, Institute of Pharmaceutical Science and Research for Girls, Swami-Chincholi, Bhigwan, Pune-Dist, Maharashtra, India

Abstract

Schiff Bases are the condensation products of primary amines with carbonyl compounds carrying imine or azomethine (–C=N–) functional group.. Pyrrolidine bearing Schiff bases developed under green reaction conditions using tamarind extract as acid catalyst. Facile green reaction conditions using tamarind extract as acid catalyst has been developed for the synthesis of diverse pyrroloidine bearing schiff's bases. Melting points were calculated using an uncorrected electrical melting point instrument. Molecular docking studies were conducted at the target protein active site using the AutoDock Vina, ChemDraw, and BIOVIA discovery studio. Pyrrolidine bearing schiff bases were synthesized using the appropriate synthetic procedure in presence of tamarind extract as acid catalyst. *In vivo* anti-oxidant activity was assessed. Compound 4a exhibited noteworthy anti-oxidant properties. Molecular docking studies at target protein PBD ID states that the compounds 4b and 4d showed good binding affinity -8.3 kcal/mol, -8.2 kcal/mol respectively in comparison to the reference compound -8.1 kcal/mol. In present work, facile method under green reaction conditions using tamarind extract as acid catalyst has been developed for the synthesis of novel pyrrolidine bearing schiff's bases. It was concluded that among all the synthesized compounds, compound 4b exhibited anti-oxidant properties and significant binding interaction at target protein

Keywords: *Pyrrolidine-Schiff bases, tamarind extract, In vivo anti-oxidant activity, molecular docking*

Presented as Oral Presentation

Assessment Of Effect Of Insomnia And Sleep Quality In Cardiovascular Patients

Scan to View online

Presented by
Dr. Anju. K. Abraham
Aditya College of Pharmacy, Aditya University, Surampalem, Andhra Pradesh, India

Abstract

A prospective observational study was conducted in a time period of 8 months in patients with diagnosis of cardiovascular diseases assessed for sleep quality and insomnia severity by using Index severity index (ISI) and Pittsburg sleep quality index (PSQI) . A total of 100 patients were included in the study. Mean age for the population was found to be 55 years. In this study male patients reporting cardiovascular complaints were found to be more than female patients. The current study shows significant correlation between insomnia and sleep quality with certain parameters like Left ventricular dysfunction, systolic dysfunction, diastolic blood pressure and stress. This study came to a conclusion that there is a need for assessment of insomnia severity and sleep quality among cardiovascular diseased patients

Keywords: *Insomnia, Ventricular dysfunction, Diastolic blood pressure, Sleep quality*

Presented as Oral Presentation

Harnessing The Power Of Flavonoids: Activating The KEAP1/NRF2 Pathway For Health

Scan to View online

Presented by
Mrs. D.Aruna Kumari
Vignan Institute of Pharmaceutical Technology, Visakhapatnam, Andhra Pradesh, India

Abstract

Flavonoids are a broad set of naturally occurring substances that are present in large quantities in fruits, vegetables, and plant-based drinks. Flavonoids have drawn significant interest because of their special capacity to activate the KEAP1/NRF2 pathway. In this paper, we investigate the intriguing interaction between flavonoids and the KEAP1/NRF2 pathway, revealing the pharmacological effects of flavonoids. NRF2 is released from KEAP1 by flavonoids like quercetin, hesperidin, and EGCG, which then translocates into the nucleus and activates antioxidant response elements (AREs), exhibiting a different method of action. Enhanced antioxidant and detoxification pathways are released as a result of this NRF2-mediated activation of cellular defense mechanisms. The pharmacological effects of flavonoid-induced KEAP1/NRF2 activation span a wide range of health advantages, including the reduction of inflammation and oxidative stress as well as the risk of developing chronic diseases. The potential of flavonoids as a natural defense system for preserving cellular health and enhancing general wellbeing is highlighted by their multiple effects in altering the KEAP1/NRF2 pathway.

Keywords: *Flavonoids , KEAP1/NRF2 pathway, antioxidant response elements*

Presented as Oral Presentation

Neuroprotective Effect of Morin Hydrate and Gemigliptin against Parkinson's disease

Scan to View online

Presented by
Ms. Diksha Shinde
Assistant Professor, DKSS Institute of Pharmaceutical Science & Research for Girls, Swami-Chincholi, Bhigwan, Pune, Maharashtra

Abstract

This study aimed to determine the neuroprotective effect of Morin hydrate and Gemigliptin in reserpine and rotenone-induced parkinsonism. Reserpine (1 mg/kg s.c.) was utilized to produce orofacial dyskinesia and rotenone (1.5 mg/kg i.p.) to induce Parkinsonism, also it causes increased vacuous chewing movements, tongue protrusions, and decreased locomotor activity. Morin hydrate (50 and 100 mg/kg) and Gemigliptin (50 and 100 mg/kg) treatment resulted in dosage-dependent substantial reductions in VCM and TP. Both drugs increased locomotor activity significantly. Rotenone administration to rats resulted in a significant reduction in latency to fall off the Rotarod and a decrease in nose poking in the hole board test. Drug treatment resulted in an increase in latency to fall off the rotarod and an increase in nose poking. Increased lipid peroxidation while decreasing levels of self-protective antioxidant enzymes such as catalase, glutathione, and superoxide dismutase in the brain. The combination of drugs reversed the effects of reserpine and rotenone on oxidative stress indicators, improving oxidative stress. Morin hydrate and Gemigliptin were found to have a protective effect against reserpine-induced orofacial dyskinesia and rotenone-induced Parkinsonism. The use of these medications may have a therapeutic potential for Parkinsonism

Keywords: Morin Hydrate, Gemigliptin, neuroprotective effect, Parkinsonism

Presented as Oral Presentation

Preparation And Evaluation Of Parenteral Delivery Formulation Containing Acyclovir

Scan to View online

Presented by
Mrs. B.Prathyusha
Gokaraju Rangaraju College of Pharmacy,
Hyderabad, Telangana, India

Abstract

Aim to develop the formulation and evaluation of parenteral delivery for formulation of acyclovir a poorly soluble antiviral drug to enhance its intravenous administration. Solubility of acyclovir in various excipients was determined. The prepared CCN AND CCP were evaluated. The formulation which showed highest entrapment efficiency 22.5% in CCN (calcium carbonate nanoparticles) and CCP the entrapment efficiency 22.4% and drug content was found in CCN 0.248(mg/ml) and the drug content also found in CCP 0.359(mg/ml).The maximum entrapment efficiency of calcium carbonate nanoparticles was found to be 22.4% (CCN-8). The maximum amount of drug content that could be loaded in the nanoparticles was estimated to be 0.719 mg/ml of nanoparticle.The entrapment efficiency of calcium phosphate nanoparticles was found to be 22.5%. The maximum amount of drug content that could be loaded in the nanoparticles was estimated to be 0.717mg/ml of nanoparticle .

Keywords: Calcium carbonate, calcium phosphate nanoparticles

Presented as Oral Presentation

A Modern Manufacturing System Facilitates Pharmaceutical Operations

Scan to View online

Presented by
Miss Yegi Sirisha
Aditya Pharmacy College, Aditya University, Surampalem, Andhra Pradesh, India

Abstract

Abstract: The "lean manufacturing" ideology in pharmaceutical operations is primarily concerned with reducing or eliminating waste and increasing production with enhanced safety and efficacy. By implementing the four important lean principles like value stream mapping, just in time production, 5S, Kaisen, and maintenance and total production. Initially Value stream mapping enhances the production process by identifying and removing waste; just-in-time production focuses on promoting a lower-cost supply chain in increased demand situations; and 5s and Kaisen are tools that organizes the workspace safe and clean to workspace while also encourages step-by-step continuous improvement. Moreover productive maintenance deals with overall equipment effectiveness, lowering the cost of equipment by preventing its breakdown. Higher output with fewer resources can be achieved through lean manufacturing's ability to increase productivity and may enhance customer satisfaction by meeting customer expectations and delivering items on schedule. Costs like labour, energy, and raw material utilization can be considerably decreased by getting rid of waste and increasing efficiency. Despite the many advantages of lean manufacturing, it's important to recognize some of its possible disadvantages, including initial investment, supply chain dependence, resistance to new change, lack of flexibility, and greater workload. Companies must carefully address these issues and adopt a progressive transformation strategy in order to get success using the lean manufacturing ideology.

Keywords: *production,waste, 5S, Kaizen, supply chain, value stream mapping,*

Presented as Oral Presentation

Nanosponges-A Review

Scan to View online

Presented by
Mrs. Mamatha Kola
Gokaraju Rangaraju College of Pharmacy,
Hyderabad, Telangana, India

Abstract

Nanosponges are tiny structures that can precisely target areas in the body to release drugs in a controlled manner. Nanosponges are created by crosslinking cyclodextrin with carbonyl or dicarboxylate, nanosponges are used for drug delivery via oral, topical, and parenteral routes, and can also carry enzymes, proteins, vaccines, and antibodies. Their nanoscale, cross-linked polymer design allows them to effectively capture and neutralize pollutants through selective trapping based on size. This review covers their preparation, toxin absorption capabilities proteins , vaccines and potential in drug delivery.

Keywords: nanosponges, cyclodextrin, proteins, vaccines, pollutants

Presented as Oral Presentation

Gene Therapy

Scan to View online

Presented by
Biswa Prakash Behera
Faculty of pharmaceutical sciences

Abstract

Gene therapy is a revolutionary medical technique that involves the modification or replacement of defective genes within a patient's cells to treat or prevent disease. It holds significant potential for addressing genetic disorders, cancers, and some viral infections at their source by correcting the underlying genetic defects. Gene therapy can be classified into two main types: somatic gene therapy, which targets non-reproductive cells, and germline gene therapy, which involves heritable genetic changes. Various methods are employed in gene therapy, including gene augmentation, gene inhibition, and gene editing, with vectors like modified viruses used to deliver therapeutic genes to target cells. Recent advances, such as CRISPR-Cas9 gene editing and CAR-T cell therapy for cancer treatment, have expanded the therapeutic potential of gene therapy. Despite its promise, gene therapy faces challenges including immune responses, off-target effects, and ethical considerations, particularly regarding germline modifications. Nevertheless, ongoing research and clinical trials continue to push the boundaries of gene therapy, positioning it as a powerful tool in modern medicine for treating previously untreatable conditions.

Keywords: *Gein therapy,CAR-T cell,*

Presented as E-Poster

Tailoring treatment to individuals for lung cancer: Right patient with right therapy at right dose and at right time

Scan to View online

Presented by

Ms. Yogita Somanath Mane, Diksha Bhagwan Shinde*

Student, DKKS Institute of Pharmaceutical Science and Research for Girls, Swami-Chincholi, Bhigwan, Pune-Dist., Maharashtra, India

Abstract

The goal of personalised medicine is to develop a treatment strategy that is as distinct as the patient's condition. The research relies on identifying genetic, epigenomic, and clinical data to advance our understanding of how a person's unique genomic makeup predisposes them to particular diseases. The personalised medicine strategy is a complete extension of the conventional (One-Size-Fits-All) approach to enhancing our ability to predict which medical therapies will be safe and useful for each patient and which ones won't, based on each patient's unique genetic profile. Although personalised medicine is a relatively new discipline, it is rapidly gaining traction. It enables a physician to select a patient's course of treatment according to their genetic profile, potentially lowering side effects and raising success rates. Several medications and approved monoclonal antibodies (mAbs) and tyrosine kinase inhibitors (TKIs) that are active against the epidermal growth factor receptor (EGFR) are being considered here in the context of personalized medicine for lung cancer. For this system, positron emission tomography (PET) is the measurement method utilized. Personalized medicine has many potential advantages, such as lowering the chance of drug toxicity, boosting the advantages of the medications taken, maintaining the equilibrium of the healthcare system, and streamlining drug development and discovery initiatives

Keywords: *Personalized medicine, Lung cancer, monoclonal antibodies, epidermal growth factor regulator, and positron emission tomography*

Presented as E-Poster

Beyond The Gut: Exploring The Therapeutic Horizons Of Microbiome Targeted Therapy

Scan to View online

Presented by
Yogalakshmi R
Dr.MGR Educational and Research Institute, Maduravoyal, Chennai, Tamilnadu, India

Abstract

The human microbiome consists of trillions of microorganisms that inhabit different areas of the body, playing a crucial role in maintaining overall health and regulating numerous physiological functions. Among these, the gut microbiome is particularly important for digestion, the production of vitamins, modulation of the immune system, and even mental well-being. When this delicate microbial balance is disturbeda condition known as dysbiosisit can lead to various health issues, including gastrointestinal, neurological, cardiovascular, and metabolic disorders. Research into the composition and functions of the microbiome has paved the way for new therapeutic strategies designed to restore and preserve health. However, despite the promising potential of these microbiome-focused therapies, challenges persist, such as the inherent complexity and variability of the microbiome across individuals, understanding long-term effects, and addressing ethical concerns. Future research should aim to identify specific microbial strains and metabolites that promote health, enabling the development of targeted interventions for precise microbiome modulation. This review emphasizes the profound impact of the microbiome on health and disease, and highlights the potential for microbiome-targeted therapies to transform healthcare across multiple organ systems.

Keywords: *Human microbiome, gut microbiome, dysbiosis, therapeutic strategies, probiotics, prebiotics, fecal microbiota transplantation, microbiome-targeted therapies, health and disease, precision medicine.*

Presented as E-Poster

Synthesis Of Novel Pyridine Containing Azetidinone Derivatives And Their Biological Evaluation

Scan to View online

Presented by
Mekala Venkata Pavana Manisha
Annamacharya College of Pharmacy,
Rajampet, Andhra Pradesh, India

Abstract

This study reports the synthesis of six novel pyridine-containing azetidinones derived from Schiff bases formed by reacting Pyridine-4-carbaldehyde with substituted aromatic amines, using glacial acetic acid as a catalyst via the Grindstone technique. The Schiff bases were further reacted with benzene, triethylamine, and chloroacetyl chloride, leading to the formation of the azetidinone derivatives. Characterization was performed using IR, H-NMR, and mass spectrometry. The compounds were tested for anti-tubercular, anti-bacterial, and anti-fungal activities.compounds exhibited significant anti-tubercular activity, surpassing standard treatments. All compounds showed good antibacterial and antifungal properties compared to reference standards like Ampicillin, Tetracycline, and Griseofulvin.

Keywords: *Pyridine-4-carbaldehyde. Schiff base, Azetidinones, anti-tubercular activity, anti- bacterial activity, anti-fungal activity.*

Presented as E-Poster

Dengue Virus Infection, Etiology, Pathogenesis, Vaccines, Diagnosis, And Therapy

Scan to View online

Presented by
Abhay Mishra, Seemu Singh , Dr. Gaurav Kant Saraogi
Sri Aurobindo Institute of Pharmacy, Indore, Madhya Pradesh, India

Abstract

Dengue virus (DENV), a member of the Flaviviridae family, is a major global public health concern, especially in tropical and subtropical regions. It is transmitted to humans through the bite of infected Aedes mosquitoes, primarily Aedesaegypti. Dengue infection manifests in a wide spectrum, ranging from mild febrile illness (Dengue Fever) to severe, life-threatening conditions such as Dengue Hemorrhagic Fever (DHF) and Dengue Shock Syndrome (DSS).

Keywords: *Keywords: Dengue virus, Dengvaxia's, Reverse Transcription-Polymerase Chain Reaction, Serological assays.*

Presented as E-Poster

Hypertension: Clinical Magnification,Diagnosis,And Management

Scan to View online

Presented by
Megha Tiwari
Sri Aurobindo Institute of Pharmacy, Indore, Madhya Pradesh, India

Abstract

Hypertension, commonly known as high blood pressure, is a prevalent cardiovascular disorder that significantly increases the risk of stroke, heart attack, and other serious health complications. Its pathophysiology is multifactorial, encompassing genetic, environmental, and lifestyle factors, leading to chronic elevation in arterial pressure. Often asymptomatic in its early stages, hypertension is referred to as a "silent killer" due to its insidious progression, which makes early diagnosis crucial. The diagnosis of hypertension relies on repeated blood pressure measurements, following standardized guidelines. Additional tests, including urinalysis, blood tests, and electrocardiograms, are often performed to evaluate organ damage and rule out secondary causes. Ambulatory blood pressure monitoring is also recommended for more accurate assessments. Adherence to treatment protocols, regular monitoring, and patient education are essential for preventing long-term complications, such as heart failure, kidney disease, and vision impairment. Despite advances in treatment, hypertension remains a major public health challenge globally, with many individuals remaining undiagnosed or inadequately treated. Continued efforts are needed to enhance early detection and optimize individualized treatment strategies for better outcomes. This review emphasizes the importance of early diagnosis, patient-centered management, and ongoing research to address the complexities of hypertension.

Keywords: *Hypertension, Angiotensin-Converting Enzyme (ACE) inhibitors, Pharmacologic interventions.*

Presented as E-Poster

The Role Of Pparγ In The Pathophysiology Of Diabetic Cardiomyopathy And Heart Failure: A Therapeutic Target Or Risk Factor?

Scan to View online

Presented by

Adyasha Nayak

Siksha 'O' Anusandhan Deemed to be University, School of Pharmaceutical Sciences, Bhubaneswar, Odisha, India

Abstract

PPARγ, a nuclear receptor regulating lipid and glucose metabolism, is pivotal in diabetes management but poses complex challenges in cardiac health. While PPARγ activation via thiazolidinediones (TZDs) enhances insulin sensitivity and reduces blood glucose, it paradoxically increases heart failure risk, primarily due to fluid retention and altered fatty acid storage in cardiac tissues. This dual role of PPARγ is linked to its impact on renal sodium reabsorption, which exacerbates edema, and on myocardial cells, where it can lead to oxidative stress and lipotoxicity, worsening heart failure. Clinical trials like PROactive and RECORD report a higher incidence of heart failure with TZDs, suggesting a need for refined therapies. New strategies such as selective PPARγ modulators (SPPARMs) and combination therapies with SGLT2 inhibitors or GLP-1 agonists show promise in minimizing these adverse effects, aiming for diabetes control that protects, rather than strains, cardiac function.

Keywords: PPARγ, Diabetic Cardiomyopathy , thiazolidinediones , heart failure, lipotoxicity in myocardium

Presented as E-Poster

Pharmacogenomics In Personalized Medicine: Current Advances And Future Directions

Scan to View online

Presented by
Shajahan K
Dr.MGR Educational and Research Institute, Maduravoyal, Chennai, Tamilnadu, India

Abstract

Pharmacogenomics, the study of how genes influence an individual's response to drugs, is transforming the landscape of personalized medicine. By integrating genetic information with drug therapy, pharmacogenomics enables tailored treatments that maximize efficacy and minimize adverse effects. Recent advances in high-throughput sequencing, bioinformatics, and pharmacogenomic biomarkers have propelled this field, especially in oncology, cardiology, and psychiatry. However, challenges like gene-drug interaction complexity, ethical considerations, and clinical validation persist. The future lies in expanding genetic databases, using artificial intelligence for drug response prediction, and adopting multi-omics approaches. Pharmacogenomics promises a transformative impact on healthcare, contingent on overcoming current barriers and ensuring widespread accessibility.

Keywords:, Biomarkers, Personalized medicine, Genetic databases etc.,

Presented as E-Poster

Revolutionizing Cancer Care : A Review Of Immunotherapies, Target Therapies, And Gene Editing Technologies

Scan to View online

Presented by
Akash Dnyaneshwar Kanhe, Nikhil Bhikaji Jagdale
Sandip Institute of Pharmaceutical Sciences, Nashik, Maharashtra, India

Abstract

Cancer has seen a significant improvement with immunotherapy, target drugs, and gene editing making treatment more promising to patients around. Traditional therapies including surgery, chemotherapy and radiation though helpful pose many drawbacks and have low effectiveness against some types of cancer. Over the past several years, the progress seen in cancer has been improved by new techniques like CAR-T cell treatment, checkpoint inhibitors, immunotherapy, and cancer vaccines, gene editors – CRISPR, and nanomedicine. The advantage of these medicines is that they raise the precision and specificity of treatments, and decrease or avoid the toxicity effect in the body thereby improving the medications safety and outcome to the patients. Targeted therapies endorse the immune system to identify and kill cancer cells, and hence the treatment provide long-term results for even the last-stage patients. Such medicines focus on particular genetic keys of cancer and have helped change, particularly for once-incurable diseases, the face of cancer therapy. Another area where nanomedicine can be it is in the functioning as a delivery tool and in cancer treatment it avoids the destruction of the healthy cells, thus improving chances of treatment. This review assesses the effectiveness, challenges and future trends of these medicines, within the broader context of their importance for the development of oncology. This suggests the need for a holistic approach as well as constant investigation into the probability of its efficiency in real life practice.

Keywords: *Cancer treatment, Immunotherapies, Target therapies*

Presented as E-Poster

Synthesize , Characterization Of Novel Diazenyl Phenyl Styryl Ketone Derivatives As Anti-Inflammatory And Anti -Tubercular Agents

Scan to View online

Presented by
K.Nagalakshmi
Annamacharya College of Pharmacy,
Rajampet, Andhra Pradesh, India

Abstract

This research focused on synthesizing novel diazenyl phenyl styryl ketone derivatives using green synthetic methods. Six derivatives were developed and evaluated for their anti-inflammatory and anti-tubercular properties. Predictive analysis via the PASS ONLINE tool indicated that three derivatives exhibited good anti-inflammatory activity, while all six demonstrated significant anti-tubercular activity. *In-vitro* anti-inflammatory activity was assessed through a protein denaturation assay, comparing the derivatives (2c, 2d, and 2e) to the standard drug Diclofenac, with all three showing comparable effectiveness. For anti-tubercular activity, the Microplate Alamar Blue Assay (MABA) was used against Mycobacterium tuberculosis, revealing that derivatives 2b and 2e had excellent activity, matching standard drugs like Pyrazinamide and streptomycin. Overall, the study presents promising new compounds with potential therapeutic applications in treating inflammation and tuberculosis

Keywords: *Phenyl styryl ketone derivatives, Anti-inflammatory activity, Anti-tubercular activity, Microplate Alamar Blue Assay (MABA), Mycobacterium tuberculosis*

Presented as E-Poster

Doxil: A Nanotechnology Driven Cancer Therapy

Scan to View online

Presented by
Bhabajit Patnaik
Siksha 'O' Anusandhan Deemed to be University, School of Pharmaceutical Sciences, Bhubaneswar, Odisha, India

Abstract

The poster "Doxil: A Nanotechnology-Driven Cancer Therapy" presents the innovative application of nanotechnology in cancer treatment through Doxil, a liposomal formulation of doxorubicin. Doxil enhances drug efficacy, reduces side effects, and increases drug circulation time compared to traditional doxorubicin. Key benefits include reduced cardiotoxicity, improved patient outcomes, and targeted drug delivery. The poster highlights Doxil's pharmacokinetics, including prolonged circulation and targeted delivery, as well as its FDA-approved applications in ovarian cancer, multiple myeloma, and Kaposi's sarcoma. Despite its advantages, Doxil has side effects like hand-foot syndrome and infusion reactions. The conclusion emphasizes Doxil's role in improving cancer therapy.

Keywords: *Cancer, Doxil , Ovarian Cancer, Myeloma, Therapy*

Presented as E-Poster

Enhancing Solubility: Innovative Techniques for improved Bioavailability

Scan to View online

Presented by
Ms. Kale Sushma, Ms. Kolekar Sandhya*
**DKKS Institute of Pharmaceutical Science and Research for Girls, Swami-Chincholi, Bhigwan-413130, Pune-Dist., Maharashtra, India*

Abstract

Bioavailability is a critical factor in the efficacy of pharmaceutical compound, directly influencing the therapeutic outcomes of orally administered drug. Poor bioavailability often results from low solubility, poor permeability, or rapid metabolism. This poster explores various strategies employed to enhance bioavailability, focusing on solubility enhancement techniques, permeability enhancers, and formulation innovations. Key solubility enhancement methods such as particle size reduction, solid dispersions, and complexation, are discussed for their role in improving drug dissolution and absorption. Additionally, the use of permeation enhancers, pro -drugs, and novel drug delivery system, such as lipid based formulation and nanoparticles, are examined for their ability to overcome physiologically based to drug absorption

Keywords: *Bioavailability, Solubility, Permeability enhancers, formulations, drug delivery*

Presented as E-Poster

Therapeutic Drug Monitoring Of Antiepileptic Drug

Scan to View online

Presented by
Triksha Panwar
Sri Aurobindo Institute of Pharmacy,
Indore, Madhya Pradesh, India

Abstract

Therapeutic drug monitoring (TDM) of antiepileptic drugs (AEDs) plays a crucial role in optimizing the treatment of epilepsy, ensuring both efficacy and safety. Epilepsy, a neurological disorder characterized by recurrent seizures, requires long-term management with AEDs. However, the pharmacokinetics of these drugs vary significantly among individuals due to factors such as age, weight, metabolism, organ function, and genetic variability. TDM provides a strategy to tailor drug dosages for individual patients, allowing clinicians to maintain drug concentrations within the therapeutic range—thereby minimizing the risk of toxicity and treatment failure. Regular monitoring of drug plasma levels can help balance seizure control with adverse effects, especially in populations prone to pharmacokinetic changes, such as children, the elderly, and pregnant women. Despite its advantages, TDM has limitations, including the timing of sample collection and the lack of correlation between drug levels and clinical outcomes in some patients. Moreover, newer AEDs, like lamotrigine and levetiracetam, may have less need for routine TDM due to more predictable pharmacokinetics. In conclusion, while TDM remains a valuable tool in the management of epilepsy, its role should be individualized, with clinical decision-making informed by both drug levels and the patient's response.

Keywords: *antiepileptic drugs (AEDs), therapeutic drug monitoring (TDM), pharmacokinetics, drug-drug interactions, plasma, serum, saliva.*

Presented as E-Poster

Digital Twins In Pharmaceutical Research And Development:A New Era Of Precision Medicine

Scan to View online

Presented by
T K T S Krishna, Dr.Gyati Shilakari Asthana
Gokaraju Rangaraju College of Pharmacy, Hyderabad, Telangana, India

Abstract

Digital twin technology is emerging as a transformative tool in pharmaceutical research, enabling the creation of virtual models that simulate biological systems, drug interactions, and patient responses in real-time. This technology utilizes vast datasets from patient health records, genomics, and real-world data to construct individualized, dynamic digital representations. In drug development, digital twins can simulate clinical trials, predict adverse effects, and optimize dosage, reducing the need for physical trials and accelerating the path to market. By mirroring human physiological responses to therapies, digital twins offer the potential for precision medicine tailored to individual patient profiles. Beyond R&D, digital twins are incorporated into pharmaceutical education to teach students about complex biological processes and the predictive power of data-driven modelling. As digital twins become integral to the healthcare landscape, they promise to enhance the accuracy and efficiency of drug development, supporting safer, more effective, and personalized treatments. This innovation not only advances pharmaceutical research but also equips future professionals with cutting-edge skills in computational modelling and personalized medicine.

Keywords: Genomics,dataset,digital twin

Presented as E-Poster

Comprehensive Diagnostic Tools Are Utilized In The Diagnosis Of Cancer And In Customizing Treatment For Individual Patients

Scan to View online

Presented by
Ankit Singh
Amity Institute of Pharmacy, Amity University, Lucknow Campus, Nijampur Malhaur, Uttar Pradesh, India

Abstract

Patients' responses to drugs vary widely, thus it's frequently necessary to use empirical methods to determine the best course of treatment for each individual patient. Ultimately, pharmacogenomics seeks to strengthen the scientific foundation for choosing the best course of treatment and dose for individual patients by further elucidating the inherited nature of interindividual variations in drug disposition and effects. Mechanism-based methods to drug discovery and development should also benefit from these genetic insights. Numerous pharmacological targets, transporters, receptors, and enzymes that metabolize drugs contain genetic variants that have been connected to interindividual variations in the toxicity and effectiveness of various treatments. For instance, thiopurine methyltransferase (TPMT) variation causes different degradation of the often given drug 6-mercaptopurine. This particular genetics variation has important.

Keywords: *Pharmacogenomics, Oncology, Cancer therapy, Pharmacological Targets, Interindividual Variations*

Presented as E-Poster

Coral Reef Management

Scan to View online

Presented by
Baibhav Acharya
Siksha 'O' Anusandhan Deemed to be University, School of Pharmaceutical Sciences, Bhubaneswar, Odisha, India

Abstract

Coral reefs, often mistaken for plants due to their vibrant colors, are complex animal structures that play a crucial role in marine ecosystems. These underwater cities are home to a diverse array of marine life and provide essential services such as coastal protection and nutrient cycling. Unfortunately, coral reefs are facing a multitude of threats, including climate change, pollution, and overfishing. Research has revealed that coral reefs offer significant potential for medical advancements. Compounds extracted from marine organisms found within these ecosystems have demonstrated promising properties in treating various diseases. For example, some compounds have shown anti-inflammatory, anti-cancer, and antimicrobial activities. However, the continued exploitation of coral reefs and the degradation of their habitats pose a serious threat to the discovery and development of these valuable resources. To protect coral reefs and ensure their long-term sustainability, it is essential to adopt a holistic approach that addresses the underlying causes of their decline. This includes mitigating climate change, reducing pollution, and implementing sustainable fishing practices. By taking proactive measures to safeguard these vital ecosystems, we can not only preserve their ecological importance but also harness their potential for medical innovation and human well-being.

Keywords: *Coral reefs, Marine ecosystems, Climate change, Ocean acidification, Coral Reef Management, Coral bleaching*

Presented as E-Poster

Protein Delivery As A Novel Tool For Tumor Targeting

Scan to View online

Presented by
Ganti Meghamala
Gokaraju Rangaraju College of Pharmacy,
Hyderabad, Telangana, India

Abstract

A tumor is a solid mass of tissue that forms when abnormal cells group together. The potential of protein anticancer specialists has however to be realized owing to the numerous uncertain issues concerning their conveyance to the location of a tumor and into tumor cells. In any case, our understanding of the instrument's fundamental to the natural destiny and biodistribution of protein and peptide drugs has progressed to an organization where strategies that utilize or impact these instruments are presently accessible. There are diverse approaches that can stride the soundness, life span, and focus on peptides and proteins in the body, such as their alteration with different solvent polymers, joining into microparticulate-medicated carriers, improved penetrability and maintenance effect-based tumor focusing, and the utilization of focusing on moieties. In addition, unused approaches to intracellular medicate conveyance, including the utilization of transduction proteins and peptides, are being developed. These progresses guarantee the conveyance of a modern era of anticancer drugs.

Keywords: *Protein, Tumour targeting, Protein delivery, Microparticles*

Presented as E-Poster

Synthesis Of Some Novel Isatin Oxime Derivatives As Potential Therapeutic Agents

Scan to View online

Presented by
Y.Madhavi
Annamacharya College of Pharmacy,
Rajampet, Andhra Pradesh, India

Abstract

The study focused on synthesizing novel isatin oxime derivatives through a straightforward method involving the reaction of isatin with hydroxylamine hydrochloride, followed by treatment with chloroacetyl chloride and DMF. This process yielded 1-2(chloroacetyl)-3-(hydroxylimino) indoline-2-one, which was further reacted with substituted anilines to produce the target compounds. The synthesized derivatives were characterized using IR, mass spectrometry, and NMR techniques. Their biological activities were assessed, revealing that compounds 4a and 4b exhibited significant anti-tubercular effects compared to standards like pyrazinamide and streptomycin, while the remaining compounds showed mild to moderate activity. In antibacterial testing, all derivatives displayed less potency than ciprofloxacin against both Gram-positive (Staphylococcus aureus) and Gram-negative (Escherichia coli) bacteria. For antifungal activity, compound 4a was notably effective compared to the standard fluconazole, with the other compounds showing mild to moderate effects.

Keywords: Isatin, isatin oxime, anti-tuberculosis, antibacterial, antifungal.

Presented as E-Poster

Osteoarthritis And Molecular Signaling: Pathways Leading To Cartilage Damage And Persistent Inflammation

Scan to View online

Presented by
Solanki Hetalben
Parul Institute of Pharmacy and Research,
Parul University, Waghodia, Gujarat,
India

Abstract

Osteoarthritis (OA) is a widespread degenerative joint disease affecting over 500 million people globally. It leads to progressive joint tissue deterioration, causing significant damage. This review explores OA's epidemiology, risk factors, and key signaling pathways, including NF-κB, focal adhesion, and AMPK, which contribute to disease progression. It also examines the roles of matrix metalloproteinases (MMPs), ADAMTS/ADAMs, and PRG4 in cartilage breakdown. Focal adhesions, with Kindlin-2 and Hic-5, are critical to maintaining cartilage structure, while NF-κB and AMPK signaling play pivotal roles in inflammation and energy regulation, offering potential therapeutic targets for OA.

Keywords: *Osteoarthritis, Signaling Pathways, Pathological Signaling Pathways.*

Presented as E-Poster

Computational Advancements In Pharmacogenomics

Scan to View online

Presented by
Romisha Maurya
Sri Aurobindo Institute of Pharmacy,
Indore, Madhya Pradesh, India

Abstract

The integration of computational methodologies in pharmacogenomics has revolutionized the capacity to predict drug responses based on genetic variation. It examines the most recent developments in computational methods used in pharmacogenomics, with a focus on large-scale genetic data processing, bioinformatics pipelines, and machine learning algorithms. Drug efficacy and toxicity predictions are becoming easier because to the discovery of intricate patterns in pharmacogenomics data made possible by machine learning algorithms, especially deep learning frameworks. Computational tools also help simulate how drugs interact with targets, predict how they are processed in the body, and design new drugs based on genetic information. In education, these tools provide interactive simulations and virtual labs, helping students understand pharmacogenomics better. However, it's important to address challenges like data security and algorithm transparency to ensure the ethical use of these advancements for better patient care and pharmaceutical success. Together, these advancements hold the potential to transform clinical pharmacogenomics, improving therapeutic outcomes and minimizing adverse drug reactions in diverse populations.

Keywords: *Computational, Genomic, Drug Response, Algorithm transparency, Genome- wide association studies (GWAS), Quantitative trait loci (QTL)*

Presented as E-Poster

A Case Study Of Surgical Management And Rehabilitation, Management And Advanced Outcome Of Diagnostic

Scan to View online

Presented by
Harshit Bhawsar
Sri Aurobindo Institute of Pharmacy, Indore, Madhya Pradesh, India

Abstract

A 37-year-old male presented with a right hip fracture following trauma, confirmed by X-ray imaging. The fracture is localized to the femoral neck, a common site of hip fractures. This injury compromises the stability of the hip joint, causing significant pain and impaired mobility. Given the patient's relatively young age, the fracture likely occurred from high-impact trauma, unlike the low-energy fractures more commonly seen in elderly patients with osteoporosis. Upon evaluation, the treating orthopedic specialist recommended surgical intervention to realign and stabilize the fractured bones. Two primary surgical options are considered: Open Reduction and Internal Fixation (ORIF) or partial/total hip replacement. ORIF involves repositioning the bone and securing it with screws or plates to promote healing. In cases of severe joint damage, a hip replacement may be necessary to restore joint function and prevent long-term complications such as arthritis or avascular necrosis. Postoperative recovery will include a structured rehabilitation program focused on restoring mobility, strength, and range of motion. The success of the surgery and recovery process will depend on several factors, including the severity of the fracture, the surgical approach, and the patient's adherence to rehabilitation protocols. Early surgical intervention, followed by physiotherapy, offers a favorable prognosis, allowing the patient to regain functional independence and minimize long-term complications.

Keywords: *Right hip fracture, femoral neck fracture, ORIF, hip replacement, trauma, surgical intervention, rehabilitation*

Presented as E-Poster

Antidiabetic Potential Of Hydro-Ethanolic Extract Of Polygonum Plebeium On Alloxan Induced Diabetic Rat

Scan to View online

Presented by
Mona Motallebi, Durga Madhab Kar, Bipin Bihari Panda
Siksha 'O' Anusandhan Deemed to be University, School of Pharmaceutical Sciences, Bhubaneswar, Odisha, India

Abstract

The objective of this study was to evaluate the antidiabetic potential of hydro-ethanolic extract of P. plebeium whole plant in alloxan-induced diabetic Wistar rats. Wistar rats weighing between 100 and 150 g were used for the study and diabetes was induced using alloxan monohydrate (150 mg/kg) intraperitoneally. The animals were treated with aqueous ethanolic extract of P. plebeium for 2 weeks. Blood glucose levels and body weight were then monitored. The antidiabetic potential was evaluated using alloxan-induced diabetic Wistar rat model (*in vivo*) by hydro-ethanolic extract. Phytochemical analysis of the hydro-alcoholic extract was done. Rats were distributed in to 4 groups. First: the normal control group; second: the diabetic control group(alloxan); third: the diabetic group which received hydro-ethanolic extract of P. plebeium; and fourth: the diabetic group which received the standard drug Glibenclamide (5mg). The phytochemical analysis revealed the presence of alkaloids, tannins, saponins, phenols, proteins, carbohydrates, gums, mucilages as secondary metabolites. This study suggests that the hydro-ethanolic extract of P. plebeium whole plant possesses a potent antidiabetic effect and may potentially be used to treat diabetes and associated complications.

Keywords: *P.plebeium, phytochemical, anti-diabetic, alloxan, phenols*

Presented as E-Poster

Targeted Delivery Of Hyaluronic Folic Acid Conjugate Decorated Cubool Jobs In The Management Of Small Cell Lung Cancer

Scan to View online

Presented by
Pramod Radhakisan Dengale
Amrutvahini College Of Pharmacy,
Sangamner, Ahmednagar, Maharashtra,
India

Abstract

This study aimed at the development of hyaluronic acid-folic acid conjugate functionalized Gefitinib cubosomes that might be useful in CD44 and folate targeting against non small cell lung cancer to overcome Gefitinib side effects and enhance its bioavailability. The GFB- Cubosomes prepared by bottoum up approach and optimized concentration of Plurol and Kolliphor P407 using box Behnken design gives 109 nm Particle size and 84.53% Entrapment efficiency. The particle size confirmed using SAXS and entrapment confirmed using DSC and XRD. The HA-g-FA synthesized by esterification reaction and confirmed its structure by FT-IR and NMR, also its affinity towards CD44 and folate receptor studied by molecular docking. The HA-g-FA GFB-CBs had a 130.7 ± 2.92 nm Particle size, − 35.40 ± 2.76 mV zeta potential, and better drug release at different pH conditions. The architecture of HA-g-FA GFB-Cubosomes was Confirmed using TEM, HRTEM and AFM. When compared to GFB-CBs, *in-vitro* experiments revealed that HA-g-FA GFB-Cubs outperformed by significantly reducing cell viability. The DPI formulation prepared for HA-g-FA GFB-Cubs and characterized using FESEM and Aerodynamic diameter. This is the first study to show that HA-g-FA GFB-CBs had CD44 and folate targeting activity against non-small cell lung cancer.

Keywords: *Cubosomes, Lung cancer, Hyaluronic acid, Folic acid.*

Presented as E-Poster

Utilisation Of Brain Computer In Neuropharmacology.

Scan to View online

Presented by
Avanti Wakte, Shaizaan Motlekar, Jayesh Baldota.
School of Pharmacy, Vishwakarma University, Pune, Maharashtra, India

Abstract

Brain-Computer Interfaces (BCIs) acquire brain signals, analyze them, and translate them into commands for external devices, bypassing the neuromuscular system. This technology aims to restore functions for individuals with neuromuscular disorders like ALS, cerebral palsy, and spinal cord injuries, and has potential applications in rehabilitation and enhancing medical professionals' performance. Future advancements depend on improving portability, safety, and real-world functionality.

Keywords: *Brain computer interfaces, amyotrophic lateral sclerosis, cerebral palsy, electroencephalography, intracortical, robotic orthoses.*

Presented as E-Poster

Formulation Of Famotidine HCl Floating Drug Delivery System Using A Natural Polymer, Bamia Gum And Pharmacokinetic Assessment In Albino Wistar Rats

Scan to View online

Presented by
M. Sabareesh, R. Jayaraman
Shri Venkateshwara College of Pharmacy,
Ariyur, Pondicherry, India

Abstract

The primary objective of this research was to generate a floating drug delivery system (FDDS) for famotidine hydrochloride using Abelmoschus esculentus L. seed gum (Bamia gum) as the release-controlling polymer.. The FDDS formulations were prepared using various concentrations of bamia gum, along with other excipients such as drug, polymers, and gas-generating agents. The formulations were characterized for physical properties, buoyancy, drug content uniformity, *in-vitro* drug release, floating behavior, swelling index, and *in vivo* bioavailability. The formulations exhibited desirable physical properties and prolonged floating time with excellent buoyancy, good swelling index and drug content uniformity. *In-vitro* release studies revealed sustained drug release over an extended period in the range of 73.92 %-92.74 % in 12 h. The *in vivo* bioavailability studies revealed that the Area under the curve showed good bioavailability, which was approximately 201.60 times greater than that of the marketed tablet. The *in-vitro* data can depict physiological conditions that are precise duplicates of those seen in *in vivo*, based on the *in-vitro-in vivo* correlation. Therefore, Bamia gum can be considered a potential polymer for the production of floating drug delivery systems, offering improved therapeutic outcomes and patient compliance for treating gastric ailments.

Keywords: *Bamia gum; Floating Drug Delivery System; Famotidine; In-vitro release studies; In vivo bioavailability studies; In-vitro-in vivo correlation.*

Presented as E-Poster

Design And Fabrication Of Ball Mill With Sieve

Scan to View online

Presented by
Avadhut Dilip Khot
Dr. Shivajirao Kadam College of Pharmacy, Sangli, Maharashtra, India

Abstract

Abstract:
This Modified machine Focuses on the design and fabrication of a ball mill integrated with a sieve mechanism for particle size control. The ball mill, consisting of a rotating cylindrical shell filled with grinding media, is designed to reduce the size of soft, non-abrasive materials. The sieve, incorporated into the system, allows for the classification of particles, ensuring that only those below a certain size pass through. This dual-function design optimizes the grinding process by providing more precise particle size distribution, enhancing efficiency and broadening its application in various industries. A ball mill is a secondary size reduction device, used for processing soft, non-abrasive materials with a hardness of 1.5 or less. It consists of a rotating cylindrical shell, partially filled with a grinding medium like metallic balls. As the mill rotates, the balls are lifted and fall, causing particle size reduction primarily through impact. Ball mills vary in size and are versatile for different materials.

Keywords: *Design, fabrication, modified Ball mill, size reduction, impact and attrition,dual function, versetile*

Presented as E-Poster

Current And Future Perspectives On Drug Delivery In Biotechnology

Scan to View online

Presented by
Jaya Jaiswal
Amity Institute of Pharmacy, Amity University, Lucknow Campus, Nijampur Malhaur, Uttar Pradesh, India

Abstract

The area of drug delivery is maturing to be a unique and multidisciplinary field of research holding attention from drug and pharmaceutical manufacturers, medical professionals, and the industry as a whole. Improved and targeted medicine delivery modes will be able to better enhance the efficacy of being specifics and also be critical for the development of novel remedial approaches, such as the delivery of peptides, proteins, glycoproteins, gene therapy, and RNA interference. with the advent of many innovative technologies coming up that make the delivery of effective medicine easier, implantable devices, nanotechnology, cell and peptide encapsulation, microfabrication, and chemical modification have surfaced; however, several challenges have to be met when such results move from clinical settings to request operation. These include scientific development that is applicable for an implementation, specific fiscal backing due to the changed scientific policy, and compliance with the government regulations and request dynamics.

Keywords: RNA integrate , drug delivery, research

Presented as E-Poster

Remote Telesurgery Robotic Systems

Scan to View online

Presented by
Uma Maheshwari G
Dr.MGR Educational and Research Institute, Maduravoyal, Chennai, Tamilnadu, India

Abstract

This review advocates the use of telesurgery as a viable option to make the healthcare infrastructure already in place around the country even more acceptable, to eliminate problems created due to scarcity of trained medical specialists in rural areas, and to provide surgical care to places that are very difficult to reach, such as space crafts and ships. Technological advancements in telesurgery robotics allow for remote control from beyond traditional distances and specialized medical environments. Good communication is needed in telesurgery. It also requires high data rates and ultra-high URLLC. Thus, the need to have 6G technology while performing telesurgery. Real-time communication is also a necessity while the success of the performance of telesurgery will be realized. Instructions given by the doctor during telesurgery can be either vocal, teleassist, or telestrategic. Hinotori was developed by Medicaroid as a robotic-assisted surgery platform, only for the purpose of pre-clinical testing via remote surgery. Edge Medical Company, Shenzen, China, reported over one hundred animal and 30 live human surgeries. The KanGuo reported human telesurgical cases conducted with distances more than 3000 km. The Microport, China has acquired over 100 human operations at a distance of up to 5000 km. However, several problems such as cybersecurity, and legal issues still need to be overcome before implementing telesurgery successfully.

Keywords: *Telesurgery, Telesurgery robotic system, Remote surgery, 6G communication, Cyber security.*

Presented as E-Poster

Beneficial Effect Of Methanolic Extract Of Pithecellobium Dulce In The Management Of Polycystic Ovarian Syndrome And Obesity.

Scan to View online

Presented by
P.A D G Lakshmi
Gokaraju Rangaraju College of Pharmacy,
Hyderabad, Telangana, India

Abstract

Polycystic Ovarian Syndrome (PCOS) primarily affects women of childbearing age, causing irregular menstrual cycles, weight gain, and fertility issues. This study examines the methanolic extract of Pithecellobium dulce for its potential benefits in treating PCOS and related complications. Using preclinical models, the extract showed significant improvements in biochemical, hormonal, and lipid profiles in DHEA and letrozole-induced PCOS models. Histopathological findings of ovarian tissues supported these results. Additionally, it effectively reversed lipid and glucose abnormalities in high-fat diet and olanzapine-induced obesity models, highlighting its anti-obesity effects. The extract also demonstrated strong antioxidant properties by scavenging hydrogen peroxide radicals and inhibiting lipid peroxidation. Overall, Pithecellobium dulce appears to help manage PCOS symptoms by regulating hormonal levels and reducing oxidative stress.

Keywords: *Polycystic Ovarian Syndrome (PCOS), Pithecellobium dulce, lipid profiles in DHEA, high-fat diet, antioxidant.*

Presented as E-Poster

Green Synthesis Of Iron Nanoparticles, Characterization And *In vivo* Evaluation Of Antioxidant Activity Of *Grewia Asciatica*

Scan to View online

Presented by
Dr.M.Prathibha Bharathi
Gokaraju Rangaraju College of Pharmacy,
Hyderabad, Telangana, India

Abstract

Nanoparticles are synthesized by employing various metallic compounds among which Iron nanoparticles are most favorable for their formation, characterization and invitro examination of biological activities like *In vivo* antioxidant activity. An environmentally safe and non-hazardous methods for applied for synthesizing nanoparticles with plants and is known as "Green synthesis"The main objective of this study is to prepare Iron nanoparticles with Grewia asciatica followed by the characterization of synthesized Iron nanoparticles by particle size analysis zeta potential UV–visible and FTIR spectroscopy.The analysis of particle size, zeta potential, UV-Visible and FTIR spectrum was determined and the Data was put into statistical analysis.The particle size of the Iron nanoparticles produced are in the range of 90 to 110 nm and the value of the zeta potential is -19.4mV, the particle size and zeta potential measurements have showed that the biosynthesized nanoparticles have a greater stability. The analysis of UV-Visible and FTIR spectrum revealed that the maximum absorbance of Iron nanoparticles was observed at 321 nm and C=C stretching vibrations in alkenes and -OH stretching vibrations in phenol compounds and alcohols was noted. The antioxidant activity (*In vivo*) of Iron nanoparticles of , Grewia asciatica was examined using the Hydrogen peroxide radical scavenging activity and the Iron nanoparticles have showed the IC50 value as 60% and when compared with that of standard ascorbic acid value of IC50 as 48%.

Keywords: *Green synthesis, Iron nanoparticles , Grewia asciatica, FTIR. UV visible*

Presented as E-Poster

Synthesis And Pharmacological Evaluation Of Novel Salicylic Acid Fused 1,3,4-Oxadiazole Derivatives

Scan to View online

Presented by
T.Chaithanya
Annamacharya College of Pharmacy,
Rajampet, Andhra Pradesh, India

Abstract

The Four novel salicylic acid fused 1,3,4-Oxadiazole derivatives were synthesized through a series of reactions starting with the esterification of salicylic acid using Ethyl-2-hydroxy benzoate. This was followed by the formation of 2-Hydroxybenzo hydrazide by refluxing the ester with hydrazine hydrate. The next step involved treating this hydrazide with substituted carboxylic acids and phosphorous oxy trichloride (POCl3) under microwave irradiation to yield the desired 1,3,4-Oxadiazole derivatives.

The synthesized compounds were characterized using various spectroscopic methods and were screened for anti-inflammatory and antioxidant activities. Some derivatives demonstrated notable anti-inflammatory and antioxidant effects.

Keywords: *Esters, hydrazides, 1,3,4-Oxadiazole derivatives, anti-inflammatory activity, antioxidant activity.*

Presented as E-Poster

The Future Of Pharmacy: Ai,S Influence On Practice And Pharmacovigilance

Scan to View online

Presented by
Pankaj Abhange
Parul Institute of Pharmacy and Research, Parul University, Waghodia, Gujarat, India

Abstract

Artificial intelligence (AI) is transforming pharmacy practice and pharmacovigilance by improving medication management, enhancing patient safety, and optimizing workflows. In pharmacy practice, AI supports pharmacists in inventory management, demand forecasting, and identifying drug interactions, enabling personalized treatment plans tailored to individual patients. It also aids in monitoring patient adherence to medications. In the area of pharmacovigilance, AI streamlines the analysis of data from various sources to quickly identify adverse drug reactions, thereby enhancing risk management and ensuring regulatory compliance. While challenges such as ethical issues and the need for training exist, the potential of AI to revolutionize these fields is substantial, necessitating continued research and collaboration among stakeholders.

Keywords: *Artificial intelligence, Pharmaceutical practice, pharmacovigilance*

Presented as E-Poster

Synthesis and Characterization Of Novel Phenazine Analogues For Antioxidant Activity

Scan to View online

Presented by
S.Riyaz
Annamacharya College of Pharmacy,
Rajampet, Andhra Pradesh, India

Abstract

The study focuses on the synthesis and characterization of six novel phenazine analogues using ortho-phenylenediamine and ammonium per sulfate in an acidic medium, followed by reactions with various aldehydes in methanol. The resulting compounds were evaluated for antioxidant activity using the DPPH method, showing mild to moderate effects compared to standard ascorbic acid. Additionally, selected derivatives were tested for antibacterial activity via agar well diffusion but did not exhibit significant antibacterial effects..

Keywords: Phenazine, antioxidant, antibacterial

Presented as E-Poster

Design And Optimization Of Curcumin-Loaded Jelly For Topical Management Of Mouth Ulcer"

Scan to View online

Presented by
Ms. Poonam Dashrath Dighe,
Mr.Shivanada Sanjay Korde
Amrutvahini College Of Pharmacy,
Sangamner, Ahmednagar, Maharashtra,
India

Abstract

Mouth ulcers are a common oral mucosal condition causing discomfort and pain. Curcumin, a bioactive compound derived from turmeric, has shown promising anti-inflammatory and wound-healing properties. This study aimed to formulate and develop curcumin-loaded jellies as a topical treatment for mouth ulcers. Various formulations were prepared using different concentrations of curcumin, gelling agents, and flavoring agents. The physicochemical properties, including viscosity, pH, spread ability, and stability, were evaluated. *In-vitro* release studies were conducted to assess the release kinetics of curcumin from the jellies. The results demonstrated that the formulated jellies exhibited desirable physicochemical properties and sustained release of curcumin. Moreover, the curcumin-loaded jellies demonstrated significant reduction in ulcer size and accelerated healing compared to control groups. Thus, curcumin-loaded jellies present a promising topical treatment option for managing mouth ulcers, offering both symptomatic relief and therapeutic benefits.

Keywords: *Curcumin loaded jellies, curcumin, antii-inflammatory, antimicrobial, woendhealing*

Presented as E-Poster

Cardiovascular Complications In Rheumatoid Arthritis: A Computational Approach To Risk Management And Treatment

Scan to View online

Presented by
Sneha Kahar
Sri Aurobindo Institute of Pharmacy,
Indore, Madhya Pradesh, India

Abstract

Rheumatoid arthritis (RA) is a chronic autoimmune disease that not only affects joints but also significantly increases the risk of cardiovascular complications, which are the leading cause of mortality in RA patients. Traditional clinical approaches focus on managing joint inflammation and autoimmune responses, but emerging evidence suggests the need for a more comprehensive strategy to address cardiovascular risks. This study presents a computational approach to risk management and treatment of cardiovascular complications in RA, integrating clinical data with advanced machine learning models. The models leverage patient demographics, clinical biomarkers, and treatment histories to forecast the likelihood of cardiovascular outcomes, offering a tailored approach to patient management. Additionally, our computational models explore the efficacy of current treatments, such as Disease-Modifying Anti-Rheumatic Drugs (DMARDs) and biologics, in reducing cardiovascular risks. Simulation results demonstrate the potential of combining anti-inflammatory therapies with cardiovascular-specific treatments to optimize patient outcomes. Future work will focus on integrating real-time patient monitoring and expanding the model to incorporate genomic data for even more precise risk prediction and treatment optimization.

Keywords: *Rheumatoid arthritis, cardiovascular complications, computational approach, machine learning, risk management, personalized treatment*

Presented as E-Poster

Advanced Drug Delivery System: Nanotechnology

Scan to View online

Presented by
Ms. Gaikwad Shruti Balasaheb, Dr. Srinivas Martha*
**DKKS Institute of Pharmaceutical Science and Research for Girls, Swami-Chincholi, Bhigwan, Pune-Dist, Maharashtra, India*

Abstract

In the medicine industry Nanotechnology plays a major role. In nano suspension particle size refers to 1-1000 nm. Nanosuspension is also used for targeted drug delivery. Nano suspension is a part of Nanotechnology. Nanotechnology is a technique that helps the poor soluble drug to make a formulation. Mostly useful for the newly developed drug which are having low solubility and also show poor bioavailability. It is prove that decreasing particle size increase the drug bioavailability, solubility and dissolution. There are more advantages of Nanotechnology over conventional techniques. Formulation of BCS II drug into the conventional dosage form is a challenge that is faced by the pharmaceutical scientist. Nanosuspension is delivered through the various routes like topical, oral, parenteral and ocular. Preparation pf nanosuspension can be done by top down and bottom-up approaches such as solvent evaporation, media milling, nanoprecipitation etc. The following review articles focus on the characteristics, application, and methods of preparation, advantages and disadvantages

Keywords: *Nanosuspension, Bioavailability, BCS II, Solubility rate, Nanotechnology*

Presented as E-Poster

Computational Oncology: Advancements In Diagnosis And Treatment Of Cancer

Scan to View online

Presented by
Sakshi Jain
Sri Aurobindo Institute of Pharmacy,
Indore, Madhya Pradesh, India

Abstract

Computational Oncology is transforming cancer diagnostic and treatment by utilizing advanced computational approaches. The convergence of data science, machine learning, and bioinformatics allows for more precise analysis of complex biological data, such as genomic, proteomic, and imaging information. Cancer remains the biggest cause of death worldwide, accounting for approximately ten million till year 2022.Early diagnosis allows for less aggressive therapies, lowers healthcare expenses, and enhances the patient's quality of life. These techniques offer more accurate screenings, early cancer detection, and individualized treatment plans. Furthermore, computer models have aided the development of personalized medicine, which analyzes unique patient characteristics to adjust therapy tactics. These algorithms anticipate treatment responses and optimize drug. Computational tools facilitate the integration of data, providing a comprehensive understanding of tumor biology and dynamics. These innovations not only accelerate drug discovery and development but also enable real-time monitoring of treatment responses, fostering a shift towards precision medicine. It's important to address challenges like data security and algorithm transparency to ensure the ethical use of these advancements for better patient care and pharmaceutical success.

Keywords: *Computational oncology, Artificial intelligence, Proteomics, Genomics, Bioinformatics , Machine learning*

Presented as E-Poster

Synthesis Characterization And Biological Evaluation Of Some Novel Quinoline Containing 1,3,4-Oxadiazole Derivatives

Scan to View online

Presented by
Arigela Mounika
Annamacharya College of Pharmacy,
Rajampet, Andhra Pradesh, India

Abstract

Quinoline which is a versatile nucleus containing 1,3,4-oxadiazoles were synthesized by conventional synthesis. Quinoline is synthesized by using nitro aniline, aryl aldehyde and an acid. To the obtained product hydrazine hydrate is added to form schiff bases and to this different aryl aldehydes were to form aldehyde derivatives. From these derivatives 1,3,4- oxadiazoles were synthesized by using POCl3. The newly synthesized derivatives were characterised by spectral methods using IR, 'H NMR and Mass spectroscopy. All the synthesized derivatives were screened for their *in-vitro* anti-Alzheimer's activity.

Anti- Alzheimer's activity is performed by using acetylcholine esterase enzyme. Results of the activity revealed that some of the derivatives showed potent anti-Alzheimer's activity and some other showed mild to moderate activity when compared to reference standard.

Keywords: *Quinoline,1,3,4-oxadiazoles,aromatic aldehyde, anti- alzheimers activity.*

Presented as E-Poster

ABOUT THE SPONSOR

This National Conference on "Computational Advancements In Research And Education For Pharmaceutical Excellence" (CARE 2024) stands as a testament to the pioneering spirit of Padma Bhushan Dr. K.I. Varaprasad Reddy garu, whose visionary leadership revolutionized India's biotechnology landscape. As the founder of Shantha Biotechnics Limited, his journey from an electronics engineer to a biotechnology pioneer exemplifies the interdisciplinary approach that this conference celebrates.

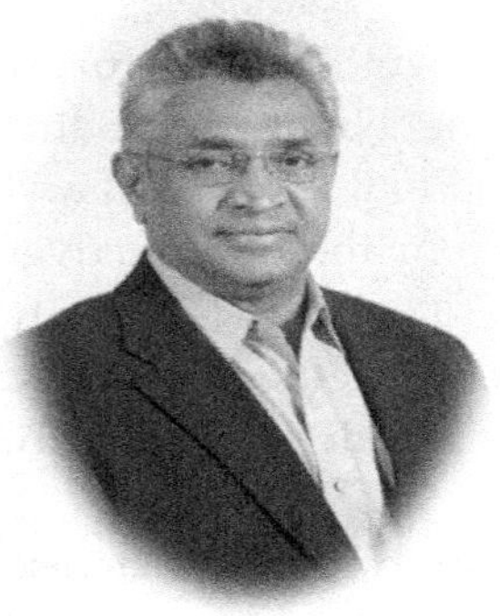

His remarkable achievement in developing India's first indigenously produced recombinant hepatitis B vaccine, Shanvac-B, in 1997 marked a watershed moment in Indian pharmaceutical history. His response to skepticism about India's capabilities at a 1990 WHO conference in Geneva transformed into a mission that not only proved India's technological prowess but also made life-saving vaccines accessible to the common man.

This annual conference, generously sponsored by him, brings together experts in computational pharmaceutical sciences, reflecting his commitment to advancing scientific research and innovation. The conference addresses cutting-edge developments in computational drug design, AI-driven pharmaceutical research, and digital transformation in drug development – areas that align with his vision of making India self-reliant in pharmaceutical innovation. The event's focus on computational approaches in pharmaceutical sciences honors his unique background in electronics engineering and computer science, combined with his groundbreaking work in biotechnology. His multidisciplinary expertise, from defense science to industrial development and ultimately to biotechnology, serves as an inspiration for conference participants to explore innovative intersections of technology and pharmaceutical sciences.

His contributions, recognized through the Padma Bhushan award and multiple honorary doctorates, extend beyond business success to encompass social responsibility and cultural enrichment. His support for yoga training and publication of works on art, literature, and music through Haasam Publications demonstrates the holistic approach to development that this conference seeks to promote. We celebrate this two-day national conference, not just for scientific advancement but also to remember the spirit of determination and innovation. His journey from Papireddy Palem village to becoming a global leader in biotechnology continues to inspire the next generation of pharmaceutical scientists and researchers. The conference serves as a platform for sharing knowledge, fostering collaboration, and advancing the field of computational pharmaceutical sciences, carrying forward Dr. KI Vara Prasad Reddy's legacy of making India a global leader in pharmaceutical innovation while ensuring accessibility and affordability for all.

Made in the USA
Monee, IL
04 November 2026

67374727R00164